The
Secret
Midwife

The
Secret
Midwife

Life, Death
and the Truth
about Birth

JB

First published in the UK by John Blake Publishing
an imprint of Bonnier Books UK
4th Floor, Victoria House,
Bloomsbury Square,
London WC1B 4DA
Owned by Bonnier Books
Sveavägen 56, Stockholm, Sweden

www.facebook.com/johnblakebooks 🅕
twitter.com/jblakebooks 🆇

First published in hardback in 2020
This paperback edition published in 2021

Paperback ISBN: 978-1-78946-457-3
Ebook ISBN: 978-1-78946-253-1

Print

Tex

The right of The Secret Midwife and Katy Weitz to be identified as the
authors of this work has been asserted by them in accordance with the
Copyright, Designs and Patents Act 1988.

Every reasonable effort has been made to trace copyright-holders of material
reproduced in this book, but if any have been inadvertently overlooked the
publishers would be glad to hear from them.

John Blake Publishing is an imprint of Bonnier Books UK
www.bonnierbooks.co.uk

I dedicate this book to your neighbour and the man who lives at number 34 – you know the one, the guy with the loud Honda. To your hairdresser, boss, friends and family. I dedicate it to your favourite celebrity, your husband or wife, your mother and father, your florist, newsagent, and the guy who just strolled past your house ten minutes ago walking his dog.

I dedicate it to your children, their teachers and the workmen at their school fitting a new light above the whiteboard in Class 2B. I dedicate it to the airline pilots who took you for a week's holiday to Ibiza in 2001, the hotel receptionist who checked you in and the girl from Exeter who lay opposite you by the pool and kept eyeing up your boyfriend on your first day in the sun.

But most of all, I dedicate it to you.

You see, all these people were born – every single one of them; we all are. And due to the miracle of life, people will continue to be born until the sun stops shining and the oceans dry up. So without them and without you, mine – and the jobs of thousands of other midwives – simply wouldn't exist.

So please accept this as a thank-you for giving me the best job in the world.

The events, situations and people in this book are real. For obvious reasons of privacy, confidentiality and to protect people's identities, I have had to make certain changes. I have altered the identifying features and aspects of some people, departments and NHS Trusts that I have come into contact with over the last twenty years. I have also had to protect myself.

However, make no mistake that this is a true account of working within NHS England's midwifery services at a number of NHS Trusts throughout my career to date. This is what really happens behind the closed curtains and locked doors of maternity units throughout the country. This is what it's like to be a modern midwife. This is what it's like to be me.

THE SECRET MIDWIFE
@SecretMidwife

Contents

Acknowledgements

Thanks to my amazing husband. No matter what we have been through, how dark my days got, or how I began to change, you never stopped loving me. Without you, this adventure would never have happened. I love you.

Thank you to my amazing co-writer Katy Weitz for her ability not just to write and listen, but to piece together the jigsaw that are my memories and then make it into something truly special.

My agent Andrew Lownie also deserves a place on this page. So, Andrew, thank you and best wishes.

My editor Ellie Carr, and the rest of the team at John Blake and Bonnier Books UK. Without their passion and hunger for my story, this book simply wouldn't exist. Thank you, thank you, thank you.

And lastly, but by no means least, I would like to thank the mystery of this universe for giving us love, laughter and wine. Life has taught me that so long as you have at least two of those, you can get through absolutely anything.

Introduction

I walk into the room and the woman on the bed gives me a hard stare.

'Well, *you* can't be the midwife,' she snaps irritably.

'I am,' I say with a smile. 'Nice to meet you. I'm Philippa, but you can call me Pippa.'

'Pippa? Are you even old enough to be a midwife?' she goes on, unconvinced. *Okay, deep breath. This one is going to be a little tricky.*

'I am indeed,' I say, picking up the notes on the end of the bed to have a quick scan of where she's at. It's Emily's first baby, she's 4 cms dilated and she seems to be progressing well. So far, so good – except she hasn't exactly taken to me. I give her what I hope is my most winning smile.

'How old are you? I bet you haven't even any children of your own. How can you understand what I'm going through?'

'I may be young, but I've already delivered tons of babies, so, don't worry, you're in good hands. You're going to be just fine. Trust me.'

The problem is, I'm twenty years old and she's scared. Quite rightly. It isn't easy, this childbirthing business, but I'm calm, relaxed and professional. I can't change my age. All I can do is try to change her mind. She doesn't know what I'm capable of yet, but I'm determined to win her round.

Emily's husband Don is sat at her bedside, nervously clutching a water bottle. I introduce myself and he offers a warm smile. Now I start to take Emily's blood pressure and she asks me sharply: 'What's that for?'

'It's a blood pressure monitor. I'm just going to take a look at your blood pressure.'

'Why?'

'Just making sure everything is nice and normal – not too high, not too low.'

'Why?'

'Well, it can make a difference to your labour if your blood pressure is too high. It increases a little during labour, so we'd expect it to be higher, but not too high or that could place extra stress on your heart and kidneys. But you're absolutely fine, so no need to worry.'

Phew. This is like a police interrogation.

'So, this is your first baby, is it? Have you got the baby's room ready?' I ask, quickly changing the conversation as I put Emily on the monitor to see her baby's heartbeat.

Emily sighs and rolls her head away from me.

'Yes, it's our first. We're nearly there with the house but, my God, it's been an uphill struggle!'

'You can say that again,' Don scoffs.

'You see, we bought this lovely old farmhouse in June last year. Beautiful place, my dream location, stunning views, loads of room for the dogs to run around – we have three Labradors – but it needs a lot of work, you know?'

I nod and smile. They are obviously very well-off – I could never afford a massive house in the country with three dogs – but it's good to get her talking while I monitor her baby's heartbeat. It also gives her less time to snap at me, and a little time to find out about her and her interests. She is talking animatedly about her house troubles, and I'm wearing my most interested smile, but, to be honest, the heart trace is not great. We usually like to see a nice, uniform but jagged line – kind of like a mountain range with no spaces or big dips. Emily's baby is showing a trace that is far more pronounced than usual. It's not exactly pathological but it's not comfortably within the normal parameters either.

No need to mention it just yet. I don't want to worry her. She is already fairly anxious and my job is to make her feel relaxed and comfortable, not to add to her worries. Now Emily closes her eyes and grits her teeth as a contraction comes on.

'Hand! Hand!' she puffs, and Don gives his hand for her to squeeze. She grabs the Entonox, and I note that so far she's only had gas and air, which is great. It means she's coping well with the pain, and that's a relief because, with a trace like this, I certainly wouldn't give her anything stronger.

'That's right, nice big breaths,' I whisper. 'You're doing really well, Emily.'

For a few seconds, there is silence in the room as Emily screws up her face and braces herself against the wave of pain that rolls over her. A distant wail down the corridor reminds me that we have four other birthing women on the ward tonight. I watch the second hand of my fob watch to count the length of her contraction, then I see her whole body unclenching as the pain passes and, without seeming to take a breath, she starts speaking again.

'But the builders couldn't start work till last September, and then we had problems with the planning and, oh, just endless interruptions. We couldn't get hold of the right plate glass for our downstairs windows. Then, when they arrived, they were the wrong size . . . yada yada yada . . . so, our room is finished, the baby's room is done, we've got no kitchen and the stairs haven't been put in yet.'

'No stairs? How do you get up and down, then?'

'A ladder.'

'A ladder? How are you going to manage your new baby with a ladder?' I say, laughing, although a little worried.

'Oh, we'll cope.' Emily dismisses my concern. 'I'm just furious about the delays, but then, what did I expect when I took on a seventeenth-century barn in the middle of nowhere?'

'With a listed roof!' Don adds.

'With a listed roof!' Emily repeats. 'Can you imagine? A bloody listed roof!'

They both shake their heads at the ridiculousness of their roof. I don't ask. I don't need to know what a *listed roof* is right now. The no stairs bit does worry me a little, but Emily seems like a formidable character – just the sort of person who would enjoy the challenge of getting up and down a ladder with a tiny infant in her arms.

I'm still not happy with the CTG trace, so I pull in the Labour Ward Coordinator (LWC) to take a look at the monitor.

'This is Angela.' I introduce Emily to the Coordinator. 'She's going to have a little look at the CTG for you.'

'Why? What's wrong with it?'

Introduction

'Nothing's wrong. It's just that we need to make sure the baby's not in any distress and the CTG tells us that.'

It's a fine line to walk when you're calling in a second pair of eyes. You don't want to worry the mum but, at the same time, you want her to feel she's getting the best possible care. We are a team, after all, and if there's any sort of problem, we rely on each other to be there at the moment we need them. This isn't an emergency, but I need Angela to be aware of the situation. Fortunately, Angela is such a pro she gives out nothing but good vibes.

Her Caribbean accent pours like honey over the anxious parents-to-be: 'Well, now, let's have a look here, shall we? How are you doing, Mum? Are you feeling alright? And Dad? Are you happy? Have you got everything you need? Good. I'm just going to take a quick look at your baby's heartbeat. Is that alright?'

Emily already has the sensor pads on her belly, which are attached to her waist on an elasticated belt, so now Angela looks at the foetal heart trace printing off on the monitor.

'Mmmm. Yes, that all looks fine for now,' Angela says. 'Nothing at all to worry about. Let's keep monitoring you and I'll be back in a short while to see how you're getting on.'

Over the next couple of hours, the contractions increase in strength and intensity and Emily is now 6 cms dilated. It's slow-going, and she's becoming more demanding by the hour.

'Get me some water! I need water!' she erupts at one point. I look at Don, who is staring straight back at me. *Me? She's talking to me!* So, I get her some water while Don rubs her back. She's wincing in pain and Don's rubs don't seem to be working.

'Oh no! Not there. *Tsk*. Get your bloody hands off me!' she barks at him.

'Is it lower back pain?' I ask quietly.

'Yes,' she groans.

'Right, I'll see what I can do.' I make her a hot compress from wet towels and place these along her lower back. She sighs with relief.

'Oh, that's so much better. Thank you, Pippa.' I gesture to Don to come over and hold the towels along her back. It's always good, I find, to get the partner involved and make them feel part of the experience.

'Once they cool down, just let me know and I'll get you some fresh ones,' I instruct.

'Can't I have something more for the pain?' Emily asks.

'But you're doing so well, Emily, with the gas and air. You really don't need it.'

'I do. I do. I really bloody do!'

'Given that the baby's heartbeat needs careful monitoring, it's probably best that I don't give you any diamorphine. I can confirm that with a doctor, if you like, but, trust me, it's best for you both if you just stick to the gas and air.'

Emily eyes me sceptically. She's still not 100 per cent convinced that I'm the right woman for the job. And though she doesn't explicitly ask me to get the doctor, I know it's probably the only way to put her mind at ease. Thankfully, and somewhat unusually, the registrar is available to attend almost straight away.

'Emily, this is Dr Hadid.' Dr Hadid is an excellent doctor, and I always feel well supported whenever she is in attendance.

On top of that, she has a wonderful bedside manner – warm and respectful – that puts all our mums-to-be instantly at ease.

Dr Hadid has a quick look over the notes and examines Emily – she is now nearly 8 cms dilated – and checks over all the previous CTGs. All the while she keeps up a steady patter with Emily, about her dogs, of all things!

'Three dogs at home! Big ones, too! Labradors are quite energetic, aren't they?' Dr Hadid murmurs while she casts her expert eye over the charts. 'I bet you have to take them out on walks a lot.'

'No, you'd be surprised,' Emily pants. 'They only need one, *urgh*, one big walk a day. But it . . . it was really good during the pregnancy. I like walking and, you know, they could definitely tell I was pregnant, couldn't they, Don?'

'They stopped jumping up on you,' Don chips in.

'That's right. They didn't jump up on me at all in the last trimester. And at night Boris and Hugo would lie next to me on the couch, with their noses on my bump. Isn't that right, Don?'

Dr Hadid laughs politely. She's not a dog person. In fact, she doesn't like animals much at all – I know because she shows zero interest whenever someone brings in pictures of their new pet.

'Well, this is all very good. All looking nice.' Dr Hadid concludes her assessment. 'I wouldn't recommend any diamorphine at this stage. It looks like you're coping well with the pain, Emily, and you're in excellent hands here with Pippa. She, as I'm sure you know already, is a first-class midwife who knows exactly what she's doing. The baby's heartbeat is fine. Baby isn't in distress; we'll continue to keep a close eye on things, but no, I don't think you need any further analgesia right now, as this could further affect the heart rate monitoring. An epidural could always be an option, though, if the anaesthetist is around.'

Emily nods quietly but says she doesn't want an epidural. I can see another contraction is coming on.

'Of course, if anything changes, I can always come back,' Dr Hadid reassures the family, but Emily is breathing hard again, closing her eyes and preparing to brace herself. I thank Dr Hadid as she leaves, and Emily scrunches up her face once more as the pain takes hold of her.

Another hour passes, and Emily and I chat happily between her contractions. I'm gradually beginning to win her over, but it doesn't stop her questioning everything I do. Or bossing me about, for that matter! During our conversation, I discover she is the finance director for a large law firm and Don is a conveyancing solicitor, so they are both very successful people in their own right. I guess they're more used to being in an office environment than in a hospital.

Emily's way of coping is to try and take control, giving me the third degree, while Don is happier to take more of a backseat. They met just two years ago, through friends, and Emily, who is now thirty-seven, was keen to start a family straight away. They were lucky to fall pregnant so quickly, she says, as she had been on the pill for almost twenty years. I look at the clock – it's been five hours, and though Emily is coming along, this is by no means a quick labour, so I decide it's time to get her mobile.

'Emily? Look, you're doing so well. You're really coming along. The towel compress will help with the lower back pain, but I think, to get you progressing a bit further along, we're going to get you up off the bed, get you moving around.'

'What? No. Why do I need to get up?' Emily objects, for a change!

I know she's tired, but that is exactly the reason we need to help things along, and the best way to get this baby out is to get her up on her feet.

'We need to get you moving to get this baby out. Don? Do you want to give me a hand? Come on!'

So far, everything I've done has been met with cross-questioning and resistance, but I'm the midwife and I know what I'm doing. I am respectful and courteous but completely determined as I help Emily off the bed and onto her feet. She resists all the way but I don't back down and, with a smile, I carry on insisting that this is the best way to progress her labour.

'Come on, Don.' I encourage her husband to take one arm as I take the other and, gently, we get Emily walking across the room. It doesn't take her long to shrug us both off and start moving around on her own, slowly but steadily, lurching from side to side as she waddles, wincing through her next contraction.

'*Ooof!*' She stops and pulls in tight, almost squatting down now. It's a good sign.

'Are you feeling the urge to push, Emily?' I ask. 'Do you want to push?'

'I–I think so.' Her voice strains.

'That's good,' I smile. 'Let's hope that means your baby's ready to make an appearance. Why don't you come over here, to the end of the bed, and then you can hold onto the bed when you want to push?' This time she does as I suggest without a word of contradiction.

Emily comes towards me and I can see in her eyes that

familiar mix of trepidation but also trust. The further along she has progressed in her labour, the further she has travelled into the realms of the unknown. Now she is in uncharted waters and all her barriers are down. This is the very first time she has given birth, and she doesn't know what's happening, so she has to have faith in me as her guide. And I do know what I'm doing. I've done it many times, and in this all-important moment, I am composed, confident and professional. I can see she's now getting the urge to push, so I encourage her to stay on her feet as gravity is helping to move everything in the right direction.

'Listen to me, Emily. You have to push down hard now,' I instruct, as she crouches down at the side of the bed. I take a quick peek at what's going on.

'It's coming!' I sing out. 'Your baby's coming. I can just see the head. You're doing so well, Emily. Keep pushing.' Don is standing next to Emily now, repeating my words, giving her encouragement.

'She can see the head,' he says excitedly. 'It's coming. Keep pushing.' I smile to myself. This is new for him, too, and he's not sure of his role in all of this, so he does what he thinks is best: he follows my lead.

I'm now on my knees, just behind Emily, as she pushes down with all her might. It's been six hours, so she's tired, but she can't stop now. Don and I both keep up the encouragement.

'Keep pushing. Keep pushing. Let's get this baby out! That's right. That's right, Emily. He's coming . . . he's coming now.'

Emily delivers her perfect baby boy into my arms, just like that, squatting at the end of the bed. It's an emotional moment. I help Don cut the cord and take a look at the little boy – he's beautiful, just beautiful! But to my mind, all babies are beautiful: tiny but perfect little human beings. If it was up to me, I'd take them all home. Now I give this little one a quick towel rub and hand him to his exhausted mother. She is beaming with pride and astonishment, as if she can't quite believe he's real.

That look! That first look between mother and child is so precious that I feel the catch in my throat. They may have been together for nine months but this is the first time they're meeting, and the bond is instant and unbreakable.

'Oh, look at you!' she whispers into the tiny bundle. Don's eyes are shining with tears. I heave myself up from the floor where I've been kneeling and see my tights are covered in blood. I'll change them later.

I leave the room, pleased for Emily and Don that I helped them deliver their baby safely, but also happy that I managed to win her round. She had started out sceptical and mistrustful, but I had done everything in my power to ensure that she felt respected, listened to and comfortable. Yes, I am only twenty, and Emily is nearly double my age, but this labour ward, this is my office, this is *my* area of expertise, and I know exactly what I'm doing.

Over the next couple of days, while Emily is being cared for on the postnatal ward, I slip in to see her a few times to make sure she's okay. They have named their son Edward Zachary Lewis, which seems like a very grand name for such a tiny person, but then I'm sure he'll grow into it. After all, he's got to hold his own against a pack of Labradors! I'm pleased to see he's latched on nicely and Emily seems to be recovering well. She's still full of questions: 'Is this normal? Is he sleeping enough? Should he have more blankets?' I do my best to answer them all. She is a new mum, after all – none of us really know what we're doing the first time round.

The following evening, Emily, Don and Edward approach me as they prepare to leave hospital. 'For you,' she whispers, as she presses an envelope into my hand. I quickly put it in my dress pocket, as I'm on my way into theatre to assist with a C-section. Later, after midnight, when I come off shift, I open the letter:

Dear Pippa,

Thank you for all you have done for us and for helping to bring our little boy into the world safely. I'm sorry I was so rude when you first came in. I couldn't have asked for anybody better to walk into my room at that moment. You handled the birth with great care and expertise and I believe you are a fantastic midwife. I'm so grateful you were the one to deliver Edward. A million thank-yous would never be enough.

Best wishes,
Emily

Fifteen years later, I still have that letter. Every now and then, as the years have passed, I've taken it out to read again, and every time it has given me the confidence and reassurance that I'm in the right job. Today, I hope I'm still that same midwife. I pick up a pen and start writing: My name is Philippa George and I'm a midwife, except today I'm not . . .

1

In At The Deep End

I knew from the age of sixteen that I wanted to be a midwife when my school sent me on a six-day midwifery taster course at our local teaching hospital. Before that moment, you would never in a million years have guessed my future profession. I was the stereotypical artsy type of girl – the girl that did well in Textiles, Art, Drama, Cookery and anything creative. Unfortunately, that didn't stretch to include Maths, English or Science. I also loved going out with my friends, possibly a little too much. You would have taken one look at me back then and said with certainty that academia definitely wasn't my strong point. In fact, if I could have studied necking Taboo shots and falling out of taxis, I'd have aced every lesson!

Luckily, I had a great group of friends and they looked after me on our wild nights out at the local club. Best of all, I had the Dad Taxi to take me home when it was all over. Dad had retired from the Force some years before, but he was still a very protective father and whenever I was having a girls' night out, he insisted on picking me up at the end of the evening. No matter what time it was – midnight, one, two in the morning – Dad was there. Maybe it was something to do with the fact that I was an only child, or maybe he'd just seen too many bad things while he was a copper. Either way, he was always there for me and managed to ignore the fact I was steaming drunk on some occasions.

'Better get yourself straight to bed,' he'd tell me if it was too obvious, meaning: don't let your mum catch you drunk! My mum ruled the roost at home and neither of us argued with her – what she said went and she would have hit the roof if she knew I was plastered. But I was blessed really. I'd grown up in a kind, loving and harmonious household and I respected both my parents enormously. By the time I was seventeen years old, I was enjoying my independence and going out with my mates at the weekend. I certainly hadn't thought about a career in midwifery until a teacher suggested there was a taster course on offer. Until that moment I'd never even held a baby!

I was, however, and had always been, slightly curious about nursing. My mother worked as a healthcare practitioner, and part of her job was to assist in theatre during operations. The stories she told me of the blood, gore and the drama that went on during surgery were thrilling, real nail-biting stuff. But up until this point I had never even set foot inside a hospital, and knew absolutely nothing about pregnancy and birth – other than the fact that my mum would have killed me if it happened to me!

The taster course was split into three main parts: we spent two days in a university, learning the theory, two days with community midwives in GP surgeries, dealing with pregnant women and seeing new mums at home, and then another two days on a postnatal ward. The university days were a big relief – since I was never very academic, I was pleased to find that the work wasn't too difficult. We learned about the process of labour and some of the midwifery jargon, which was both daunting and truly fascinating. Then I joined the community midwife in my local GP surgery, looking after pregnant mums-to-be.

The women would come into the surgery, some with rounded tummies who barely looked pregnant at all, others waddling like ducks with great bumps in front of them. We talked about how they were coping and what advice the midwife could offer to help them along. Then the midwife performed various observations, took their blood pressure and measured the bump to check that the baby was growing normally. Finally, she would use a small handheld device called a Sonicade, to listen to their baby's heartbeat. That was always a very special moment. Whether it was the first time, or if she'd heard it many times before, each woman's face transformed with joy as she heard the strong, thumping beat of that little baby inside her.

The thing is, most pregnant women have no idea what's actually going on inside them. They know their baby is growing but there's always that anxiety at the back of their minds that something could be wrong. The worry only disappears when they have real proof that the baby is okay – so when they hear the heartbeat they are flooded with relief. Scowls are replaced with genuine, natural smiles and the whole mood in the room lifts. It's like a switch has been flicked on. It was such a high to be part of that, I found myself constantly grinning with delight due to their happy vibes. When my community midwife did an abdominal palpation, to see which way the baby was lying, she got me to put my hands on the bump too. What a sensation! Barely out of childhood myself, it was exhilarating to feel the outline shape of that little life growing inside her. None of my friends or close family had babies, so I'd never spent any time around pregnant women before now. It was amazing to see this whole other side of life I knew absolutely nothing about.

The other part of the community midwives' job was to visit women in their homes after the birth. Meeting those new mums and listening to their stories of what they went through, I was enthralled. What could be more precious than to watch a baby's first breaths, first cuddle, first smile? The women put complete trust and faith into their midwives. Here we were, strangers from very different walks of life, suddenly thrown together at the most intimate, special and often scary moment of a woman's life. The bond was instant. I'd not yet witnessed a birth at this point, but I was desperate to see one, and to be that person who helped bring new life into the world.

Finally, we had our two days on the postnatal ward, helping out with women in hospital who have just given birth. Every moment was an eye-opener, an insight into this incredible process of giving birth and, thanks to the generosity of the midwives and the women they looked after, we were given plenty of opportunities to help out and get close to the new mums. In fact, a little too close on one occasion.

On my second morning, I was shadowing a midwife who had to remove the catheter from a lady who'd had a C-section. The lady was very sweet and had said she was happy for me to be there and to watch. So I paid close attention as the midwife deflated the catheter and slowly removed it, but maybe, in my keenness, I was standing a little too close because, as the tube came out, there was some tautness and then, a second later, as if in slow motion, it pinged back and flicked me in the face. *Urggh!* Someone's wee was on my face! I instantly flushed red-hot and my ears started to ring. My stomach turned over and, in that moment, I really thought I was going to faint.

'I need to go to the bathroom,' I mumbled, before racing to the toilet and washing off whatever it was that had hit me. Slowly, after making my face red from all the scrubbing, I sat on the toilet, placed my head between my legs and tried to compose myself. I must have been there a good fifteen minutes, ears still ringing, mind racing, thinking, *I can't do this. I can't do this. It's disgusting.* But after that initial wave of nausea and panic had passed, and I'd calmed down enough to stand up, I felt the urge to get straight back to the midwife I was shadowing. I didn't want to miss a thing. It makes me laugh thinking of that incident now, of how revolted I'd been at a tiny little splash of urine. Since then, I've come to realise that having close encounters with all manner of bodily fluids is a hazard of the job, and it doesn't bother me one bit.

It took just six days to convince me that I wanted to be a midwife, and by the end of that week I knew I had found my calling, my vocation. This was my future! I was so determined to fulfil my destiny that, straight after the taster course ended, I marched into my local bookshop and bought all the books I could find on pregnancy. Not midwifery books, mind, books for actual *pregnant women*.

What an idiot! I didn't care. I was hooked, and I devoured every word in those books in my bedroom at home while my Celine Dion and Motown CDs blared out of the stereo. I knew midwifery was for me, and so I set about trying to achieve my goal. After returning to school and limping through my AS levels, I applied through UCAS for a place on their next available midwifery diploma course (this was back in the days before you needed A levels to apply), at a university about an hour away from my home, and was so excited when I managed to get an interview just as the new school term was starting in September.

I arrived at the interview in my smartest clothes, nerves flooding my system. There, I met two of the other candidates – both of whom were much older than me. One was in her mid-thirties and the other was early forties (and, funnily enough, they both now work at my NHS Trust). Despite the age difference between me and the other candidates, and my nervousness, I felt reasonably confident the interview had gone well on the day, having answered all the interviewer's questions with a great deal of enthusiasm and newly acquired knowledge. But in December I got a letter to say my application had been unsuccessful.

I was devastated. This was my calling, my destiny. *How in the hell was I meant to become a midwife now?* I called the university to ask for some feedback, and to find out what had gone wrong. The interviewer was quick on the line.

'Pippa, you interviewed really well,' she said apologetically. 'But I'm afraid the interviews are scored on a points system and the others just scored higher than you, probably due to their ages and life experience.' I was still only seventeen; that was my downfall.

'Don't give up,' she went on encouragingly. 'You'll get there. I'm just sorry that on this occasion it wasn't your time, but please do apply again next year and we'll bear you in mind. '

She had been kind enough, but I felt utterly hopeless. *What am I going to do?* I despaired. I wasn't enjoying A levels, and I was so convinced I wanted to be a midwife that I knew I had to find another way to get there. So I made the decision to drop out of school and start a Health and Social Care access course at the local college.

It was awful – the worst mistake of my life – and I hated every minute. I hated the environment, I hated the work, I just hated everything about it. Unlike school, the college day was completely unstructured and, since I didn't know anybody, I felt lost and so lonely. It was the middle of January and, by the end of my first week, I was utterly despondent. Negative thoughts ran through my head like a loop tape: *I'll never achieve my dream. I'll never be a midwife. I might as well just give up now.* Then I got a call from my old headmaster. He wanted to know why I'd stopped my A levels. I burst into tears on the phone.

'I know I want to be a midwife,' I explained, 'but I failed to get on the course. And now I'm on this access course and it just feels all wrong for me. I don't know what to do. I know where I want to be, but I just don't know how to get there!'

'Right, Pippa, come back to school and pick up your A levels,' he said. 'Stick with it. Honestly, you'll be fine. Then, next year, just reapply for the midwifery course.'

It was the kick up the bum I needed, and a gratefully received Plan B. Yes, there was always next year, as he'd said. So, I went back to school the following week and picked up where I'd left off with my Biology, Psychology and Health Care A levels. At least I now had a plan to achieve my dream.

The following month I got a call from the university. One of the successful applicants had dropped out and would I like to take her place? If so, could I start in two weeks' time?

Woo-hoo! What a roller coaster! In the space of three months I'd gone from the depths of despair to utter joy, and in two weeks I would start my midwifery course. Finally, I was on the right track.

On my first day at university, I was so nervous I was practically shaking. After all, this was still only March, so most of my friends were still at school, completing their A levels. I was the only one who had started university early and I had no idea what to expect. Fortunately, all the student midwives on my course were lovely and incredibly friendly. There were twenty of us in total, and I was the youngest by quite some way. Nancy, who I carpooled with, was in her fifties, and the rest of the students were in their thirties or forties. There was only one other girl close to me in age and she was twenty-five. I was definitely the baby of the class, but it didn't seem to matter. We quickly bonded and became a tight-knit group, helping each other out when we needed it.

The diploma course was divided into two halves – practical and academic work. For the first eight weeks, we were all based at the university, learning the theory. Essays were not my thing, and every time we were set a piece of writing work, I felt wobbly and unconfident, but as soon as we were out in the community, learning the practical side of things, I was in my element. Our placements divided into three parts: the labour ward, postnatal and antenatal, and community placements. We also did shorter stints in other areas of the hospital to improve our general nursing skills.

At first, we were given community placements, seeing pregnant women, so it wasn't until eight months into the course that I actually visited a labour ward for the first time. I'd never witnessed a real birth and was still very naïve. On my very first labour ward shift, I was assigned to a mentor called Beverley, but halfway through the morning we became detached and I ended up wandering around the unit like a lost lamb, looking for her.

'Have you seen Beverley?' I asked various members of the team.

'Why don't you try in there,' one said, pointing to a closed door.

I walked into the room and there, on the bed, was a woman cradling a tiny bundle. The room was quiet and still, and the child appeared to be resting in her arms, held lightly on her lap.

'Ah, thank goodness!' she said when she saw me, her voice steady and calm. 'I've been ringing the buzzer for ages. Can you put my baby back in the fridge, please?'

'Sorry, can you say that again, please?' I said, thinking I'd misheard her.

'Can you put my baby back in the fridge,' she repeated.

My heart stopped. She'd said it so casually, like it was the most normal request in the world. *Fridge? Why would I put her baby in a fridge?*

And then I caught sight of what was hiding inside the blankets she was embracing – a very still, very pale baby. Clearly dead.

21

'I . . . uh . . .' I shakily took the cool bundle from her and she sensed my confusion.

'It's in the room back along the corridor,' she offered. I mumbled something incoherent and walked out with this stillborn infant in my arms. The coldness shocked me.

'Erm, what do I do?' I asked the first person I saw. The midwife caught the panic in my breaking voice and took over, delivering the baby back to the long metal fridge in a small side room off the corridor. I had never even imagined this place existed – a room with a large fridge and shelves just big enough to slot small bundles into. Underneath there were drawers labelled with items of baby clothes – hats, babygrows, vests and blankets – all, I now realised, for the babies who never made it.

I didn't want to see any more. I ran, the sound of blood rushing through my ears, and hid in the toilets, sobbing. I'd never even held a baby before, and on top of that I'd never seen a dead person, but here I was, my first day, and all before 9 a.m.! I just wasn't prepared for the sight of that tiny pale body with its skin peeling off, the veins visible through its translucent little face and its eyes still fused together. *Could I cope with this?* That very first day, I was considering whether midwifery was really for me.

When I was finally reunited with Beverley, I had to explain my absence from the ward. I suppose the sniffing and my puffy red eyes gave the game away.

'Oh no!' Beverley looked crestfallen. 'You should never have been sent in there. I'm so sorry, Pippa, I should have been with you. It's just that I was called away by an emergency buzzer. I'm sorry. Are you okay?'

'It was a bit of a shock,' I admitted.

In at the Deep End

'I know, I know. You should never have been put in that position, but you absolutely must not let this put you off. Yes, it's true that some babies don't make it, and we have to deal with that. Grief, loss, bereavement – it's all part of the work we do here. But it's something you get used to over time, and it's by no means the norm. I promise I'll make it up to you. Come on, I'll start by buying you a cup of tea.'

Beverley was true to her word. She looked after me so well after that incident, and she made sure my time on the unit was memorable. It was my first day on the labour ward and I'd been thrown in at the deep end. As it turned out, midwifery is full of firsts . . .

2

A Hands-on Job

You never forget your first baby.

I had thought I could take a backseat this first time, but Beverley had other ideas. Mum was fully dilated and had been pushing for forty minutes before the head started to crown.

'Right, there's no time like the present,' Bev said. 'Come here, Pippa, and get your hands on this baby's head.'

'What? Are you sure? I've not even seen a birth before. Just let me *see* one first,' I begged, panic rising inside my chest.

'No, let's do this. Come on! Just put your hands on mine.'

It was a low-risk pregnancy, which meant we were in the low-risk birthing unit. Fairy lights twinkled, music played softly in the background, and the scent of aromatherapy oils wafted round the room. The mum was doing fine – she was sitting on a low couch, leaning back against her partner, and so far, there were no complications.

'Come on, push!' Beverley prompted.

I took a deep breath and inched forwards, then I put my hands on the baby's head. It was warm and slimy, soft yet firm at the same time, like a ripe piece of fruit. I'd never felt anything like it before.

'That's right,' said Bev. 'Just get a feel for the pressure.'

Mum bore down hard, gripping her partner's hands and, gradually, the baby started to emerge. Beverley had her hands over mine the whole time, talking me through the process of descendance, the rotation of the head, and what kind of pressure to apply, until a little boy came sliding out and we heard those first amazing cries. I felt like crying, too. It was overwhelming. I'd never even seen a birth before now, and here I was helping to deliver a new life in the world.

'Has he got a name?' I asked a while later, as their little boy was being weighed.

'Jack Daniel.' Mum gave Dad a sly smile. 'Because that's what we were drinking the night he was conceived. He's called Jack Daniel Jones.'

I couldn't stop giggling. I would definitely never forget my first baby now. I left the room, buzzing and tingling with adrenaline, hardly believing what I'd just done, but also proud to feel like one of the team. It was so much to take in, I shed a few tears later. Happy tears.

'Are you alright?' Beverley put a reassuring hand on my back.

'Yeah. I'm . . . it's just . . . wow! God, that was amazing.'

'Yeah, it is, isn't it?' she laughed.

I couldn't believe that I had assisted at my very first birth. It was the biggest high of my life. And this meant I was one step closer to becoming a real midwife. Only thirty-nine more births to go before I could qualify.

A Hands-on Job

* * *

Beverley was a great mentor. She encouraged me to get stuck in at every point, pushing me to do things I was scared of and helping me overcome my limitations. I wasn't always the happy, confident midwife that I am today, and the labour ward wasn't always my second home. To begin with it was a weird, alien environment where very important doctors and midwives strode around, speaking to each other in a language I didn't always understand. I had to work hard to apply the knowledge I'd learned in university to the practical side of looking after women in a labour ward.

And I had to gain my confidence on the ward – getting used to holding my own when I was talking to doctors and other senior members of the team. They seemed so intimidating at first, but Beverley wouldn't let me hide behind her years of experience. She would turn to me whenever the doctors asked a question, prompting me to speak and offer my thoughts. It brought me out of my shell, and, over the next few months, I assisted her with dozens more births. Every day, we came across a new situation that added to my experience, skills and ability to deal with different complications. What I learned most was that this was a *team effort* – it was always exciting to help a woman give birth, but when things didn't go according to plan, the whole crew was there to help out. They were trained and experienced; everyone knew what they were doing and the whole unit worked like a well-oiled machine. I learned how to put my trust and faith in the other professionals around me and take my place as part of that team.

Though I always tried my best, it was a steep learning curve, and there were one or two occasions when I didn't quite live up to my own expectations. I was six months into my training, and working a night shift, when I was called into theatre to observe my first caesarean section. I'd read my books on C-sections, so I thought I knew what to expect. But this was the first time I had been inside an operating theatre, and nothing can quite prepare you for seeing it all up close. After I'd scrubbed up, I was told where to stand so that I was in full sight of everything that was going on, but given strict orders about what I could and couldn't touch. Everybody around me had a job, and they all worked quickly and quietly, offering information and reassuring words to the expectant mum and dad as they operated. I had one job and that was simply to observe. So I did.

I watched as the anaesthetist carefully put in the spinal.* Then they laid the woman down and inserted a catheter. This was important, since she would be numb from the waist down and unable to get up to go to the bathroom afterwards. The registrar and Senior House Officer [SHO] began to prod the abdomen with their fingers, testing to see where to make the first cut. They then went ahead and made an incision, slicing the belly from what seemed like one hip to the other, although it was probably only 4–6 inches, until they had a long, deep cut. That was just the first layer of skin. Next, they made another incision, through the layer of yellow fat, which exposed the thick abdomen muscles below. Now the registrar and consultant each put their fingers on either side of the bright-red sinews and

* A spinal is not the same as an epidural, they are actually two quite different forms of analgesia. The spinal numbs from the chest down and paralyses the lower limbs, and while an epidural numbs, too, the woman is still able to move. A spinal is given during a standard C-section, and a general anaesthetic is usually given for an emergency C-section, when there is no time to put the spinal in.

started to yank at them sideways, pulling the muscles apart. I was gobsmacked. Before this moment, I had never really considered how the muscles were moved in order to get at the baby – it turned out the answer was sheer brute force. Of course, the woman couldn't a feel a thing, but you could see from the way the doctors were straining and leaning back that they had to put a lot of strength into the job of separating those muscles, enough to make room for a baby to come out. It was fascinating but horrifying at the same time, like watching a woman being turned inside out. At that point, I started to hear ringing in my ears.

When the muscles were far enough apart, I could see the big pink sac underneath – the uterus. It was very light in colour, with small vascular veins running up and down it. My head felt fuzzy, as if it was full of cotton wool. Next, the registrar made a small incision in the uterus, breaking the waters, and a scrub nurse moved in with what looked like the head of a Hoover, sucking up all the waters around the baby. A whooshing, sucking sound filled the theatre, as the waters disappeared up the thick tube. The registrar then scooped his hands into the sac and out popped the baby's head.

I had just caught sight of the baby's body being pulled out when I felt myself starting to go. It was like a trapdoor opening beneath my feet – I was falling and there was nothing I could do about it. Within a few seconds all the strength drained from my body and I collapsed in a heap on the floor. I sensed someone at my side, and my body shifting about, until they had sat me up against the wall.

There was a strange throbbing in my head and my senses were all mixed up. I wasn't totally out of it; I could see what was happening around me, but my hearing had gone, so everything was taking place in a vacuum of silence. Someone handed me a cup of water and I sat there, on the floor in theatre, sipping water, while this woman met her baby for the first time. I couldn't have felt more like an idiot if I tried! They were sewing her up and sorting her out, and everyone was just stepping over me, ignoring the fact that one of their student midwives was in a pile on the floor. My head swam, and I felt so shaky I wasn't sure I could stand up. Thankfully, once they'd wheeled out the patient, two kindly scrub nurses lifted me to my feet and took me to the staff room, where they plied me with hot, buttered toast and sweet, milky tea until I felt my strength returning. Another ten minutes went by and I started to feel much more myself again. And then, oh God, the humiliation hit me!

'I'm so embarrassed,' I groaned.

'Don't worry about it,' one of the scrub nurses said, smiling indulgently. 'You're not the first, by any means. You wouldn't believe how many fainters we've had in that theatre.'

'Really?'

'We have SHOs walking out and collapsing in that corridor pretty much every other week. It's normal. You'll get used to it, don't worry.'

And I did. I got used to a lot of things. Every day, I worked hard to put into practice what I'd learned in university, and by midway through my second year, I'd already delivered forty babies, which was the magic number you needed to qualify. Working nightshifts had helped – babies tend to come at nighttime, so I managed to hit my target quite quickly. But it didn't matter how many babies I helped to deliver, that heart-stopping joy at the birth of new life was overwhelming every single time. At first, Beverley was with me all the way, standing at my shoulder, giving me one-to-one support and feedback, insisting I took my breaks – even if she wasn't getting them herself – looking after me, guiding me, making sure I had something to eat and drink. But the further I got into my training, the more I was left to do things on my own and manage the births without her help.

By the start of my second year, if the delivery was low risk, Beverley left me entirely alone, only popping in every now and again to make sure everything was okay. One day, I was assisting a lady who was fully dilated and was crouching on all fours, leaning over the bed, pushing. I had my delivery tray all set up. This included a soft baby blanket, a sterile sheet to deliver the baby onto, two Spencer wells (metal cord clamps), two plastic cord clamps, episiotomy scissors, cord scissors, maternity pad, five swabs (all X-ray-able), a kidney dish (for the placenta) and a small bowl used for washing down afterwards or catching wee if we need to catheterise.

I stood behind her with my gloves on, ready to catch. I could see there was a presenting part coming but I didn't know what it was. *Could it be the head?* I bent down lower to get a better look, but all I could see was a big water sac coming, like a giant white balloon. *Where was the baby's head?* I inched in closer to see if it was coming behind the water sac. *Hmmm . . . no, nothing.* I got a little closer. *Is it coming? Where is it?* Now I was just inches away, and suddenly – *WHOOSH!* The sac broke all over me. I was drenched, head to foot, in waters.

Oh gosh. Oh no.

I closed my eyes. The thick, gooey stuff dripping down

my face was meconium – baby poo! I could feel the gungey green slop dripping off my head and soaking through my scrubs. *Urgh! It was in my mouth!* At that moment the door opened and in walked Beverley.

'Oh dear!' she exclaimed when she saw me, holding a hand over her mouth to stifle a giggle. 'Oh my, look at you!'

'Erm . . . a little help here, please?' I squealed.

'Come on, Pippa.' She was laughing now. 'Let's get you cleaned up.' Beverley grabbed a handful of paper towels and wiped my face. Then she whipped off my gloves and apron and handed me some fresh ones.

'*Oooh!*' The birthing mother let out a strained groan. I knew she was pushing, so there was no time to lose. I popped my gloves back on and crouched down again. I couldn't leave her; she was delivering! And sure enough, a few minutes later, her beautiful baby girl slid out and I caught her, still covered in slimy waters and gooey baby poo.

The moment of birth is always euphoric, and, on this occasion, it had happened so quickly that both mum and her partner were caught off-guard. They gushed tears of happiness, and I too was caught up in the euphoria, practically floating on air when I left that room. I bounced off down the corridor to the nurses' station, my hair still plastered to my head and bits of goo sticking to my clothes but wearing a grin a mile wide. The two midwives at the nurses' station did a double take when they saw me.

'Bloody hell! What happened to you?' one exclaimed.

'Oh yeah. I forgot about that. I got drenched in waters.'

'Pippa, you're going to have to wash your hair,' Beverly said, as she came up behind me. 'You can't stay like that. You'll give our ladies the shock of their lives.'

A Hands-on Job

So I took a quick shower, scraped my hair back in a ponytail, changed into a fresh pair of scrubs and dived back onto the ward, ready to carry on my shift.

* * *

It's fair to say I did a lot of growing up during my three years of training. I went into the course a naïve and inexperienced seventeen-year-old, but by the time I came out at twenty, I was a different person. I'd seen a whole lot more of life and I now knew how to deal with every sort of emergency situation. It wasn't just the labour ward; the time I spent in hospital on my general nursing placements was also a real eye-opener.

As part of our course we were required to spend some weeks in different parts of the hospital, in order to improve our core nursing skills. My first placement was on the Emergency Assessment Unit, which is where patients go after they've been seen in A&E and are waiting for a bed. There I saw all sorts of different emergencies – the elderly who had tumbled down stairs, overdoses, abdominal pains, broken bones, alcoholics, stroke victims, dementia patients. Anyone, in fact, who was waiting for a bed to become available. For all these illnesses and emergencies, we were required to do general nursing work like taking blood pressure, taking blood samples, doing observations, putting in catheters, administering meds – you name it, we did it. And I loved it. Not necessarily the work; it was the different people and the unexpected nature of my day.

One woman, Estelle, brought herself in every Saturday night like clockwork, having drunk antifreeze. I wouldn't call them serious suicide attempts, more like cries for help. She was a young girl, mid-teens, and she clearly had a troubled home life. Well, it turns out that the antidote to drinking antifreeze is alcohol. So, whenever Estelle presented herself to A&E, we would have to crack open a bottle of ethanol and either give it to her pure in small doses or mixed with orange juice. It's normally given intravenously, but Estelle wouldn't let us near her with a needle, so every two hours it was my job to give her a measure of the stuff, until, by about 4 a.m. on a Sunday morning, she was as pickled as a radish.

'Feels a bit funny, getting her drunk like this,' I commented to another nurse.

'Mmm . . .' she murmured. 'Almost like she's doing it deliberately to get herself legally pissed?'

'I don't think so. I mean, for a teenager she's going to extreme lengths to get a bit of alcohol down her when she could probably just buy some alcopops from her local corner shop.'

'Yeah, but here she gets it for *free*. Just saying. I mean, she turns up every weekend and it's always the same. You'd think if she really wanted to do herself in she would have come up with another method by now.'

I wouldn't let myself get that cynical. I'd seen this poor girl admitted to ITU no end of times, and I also knew she was under the care of the mental health team. Whatever had led her to drinking antifreeze, it was a genuine crisis. She had been diagnosed with a personality disorder – only the poor thing had no support from her family. One night she was so distressed, she threw herself out of bed and landed headfirst on the floor.

That night I took her for a head scan, and we talked

until the small hours of the morning. I felt like I was part counsellor, part nurse, part bartender.

'I'm training to be a midwife,' I told her, as I poured her another shot of vodka.

'I'll never have children, me,' she slurred, shaking her head. 'I'm not well enough to ever have children.'

I thought about Estelle a lot through the years, wondering how she was getting on, how she coped since that bleak period in her teens. And then, one day, about five years ago, I recognised her name in the handover notes. She had given birth the night before. I went onto the ward to see her and, despite the labour, she looked incredibly healthy – a world away from the skinny, troubled teenager I had helped to treat years earlier.

'Do you recognise me? We've met before,' I told her. 'You told me you'd never have a baby, and look, here you are!'

'Oh my God! I can't remember you. I'm really sorry.'

'I'm not surprised. You were sozzled on vodka most of the time. Anyway, it's good to see you.'

Until that point I had led a relatively sheltered life. My parents were both hard-working people who'd protected me from the more distressing aspects of the grown-up world. If there were crises among our family or friends, I wasn't told about them. But on the Emergency Assessment Unit, I saw people on the very edge, and it opened my eyes in a way I'd not experienced before.

For instance, one young lad of twenty, Adam, had taken an overdose of painkillers, and was brought in by his father and brother, who were both beside themselves. Adam was unconscious and needed his stomach pumped. While we were getting his bed sorted out and everything ready, the dad went out for a cigarette. That's when Adam's brother confided in me.

'He's a secret gambler,' he whispered. 'Dad knows nothing about it. He's too ashamed to tell him. He's addicted to cocaine, too. It's like a double life. To Dad, he's the blue-eyed boy who can do no wrong, but that's just what he wants him to see. Adam's in trouble. He's racked up huge gambling debts. That's why he did this. He couldn't see a way out.'

I felt so sorry for them all. I just hoped that after Adam's desperate actions, he could find a way to be honest with his father and ask for help.

* * *

I spent four weeks on the Emergency Assessment Unit in total, followed by six weeks on the gynaecology ward, a couple days on the respiratory ward, then a week with the diabetic team. At the beginning of my third year I was sent back to the labour ward to complete my training.

'So, how was it?' Beverley asked. 'Hated every minute, did you?'

'God, no! I loved it. All of it!' I enthused.

'Well, that makes a change. Most of my students find their placements a real drag, taking them away from the labour ward and all the babies.'

'Not me. I thought it was so interesting. Honestly, Beverley, you'll never believe the things I saw!'

It was true, I was glad to be back on the labour ward but, from here, things got much tougher.

3

True Knots &
Bacon Rolls

Jessica was thirty-six weeks pregnant and had gone for a routine midwife's appointment at her GP practice, only to be given the worrying news that her midwife couldn't hear the foetal heartbeat. Panic-stricken, she was immediately sent to the hospital for an ultrasound scan where it was confirmed – while Jessica lay there alone in that dark room, the ultrasound gel still cool on her belly – that no heartbeat could be detected. The baby was stillborn. If that wasn't devastating enough, it was then explained that she would need to be booked in for a procedure called an induction so she could give birth naturally.

It was the first time I was put in charge of caring for a woman delivering a stillborn and, I have to admit, I was scared. It was now my third year of training. Although I'd gained lots of experience delivering live, healthy babies, I'd never actually supported a woman giving birth to a baby knowing they hadn't made it. I had been protected from this part of the job until now. In the first year, we had learned about the normal aspects of labour. In the second year, we were introduced to complications and interventions, like forceps, which were still relatively normal. But now it was my third year and I was being asked to deal with some of the more challenging situations a midwife might have to face.

Jessica and her husband Adam arrived on the ward at the start of my nightshift and, as you might expect, they were both very emotional. After Jessica's last scan – the one confirming the devastating news of the intrauterine foetal death – she was given the drug Mifepristone, a medication that stops pregnancy hormones and is often used in abortions. Jessica and Adam then had to return home for twenty-four hours before coming back in for another drug called Misoprostol, that starts off labour.

I did my best to make a bad situation as good as it possibly could be, but I felt the weight of their pain. Far from the joyous occasion she had been expecting for the birth, this was going to be an horrific and painful struggle. They were devastated. And, naturally, I felt terrible for them. I'm only human, after all, and I've got my own emotions. But I had to remain as professional as I could – I had only one chance to get this right. Whatever I did, they would remember this night for the rest of their lives.

To begin with, Jessica was quiet, seemingly lost in her pain and confusion, occasionally hugging Adam and shedding a few tears. Then, after a couple of hours, she started to open up to me. We didn't talk about the baby straight away – she didn't seem to want to. Instead, we talked about films, music, TV shows – you name it, we gabbed about it. We talked about their jobs: he worked for building company; she was a teacher. We had long conversations about anything and everything, just to take her mind off what she was going through. Occasionally, just occasionally, she'd stop speaking and burst into tears. Then a sad silence would descend on the room while she tried to re-erect her façade of strength.

A few hours in, she said to me: 'I think the worst part is that I didn't know. I mean, I was just going about my normal day, thinking about what I was going to cook that night, and getting the painting finished in the baby room. And he wasn't even alive any more. How could I have not known?'

'I suppose nothing changed,' I said. 'Your body doesn't know what's happened to your baby. You are still pregnant, so it's still producing all the hormones. And it might have happened really quickly before the appointment.'

'I thought he had moved the night before. I really did. I mean, if he went quiet for a little bit, I noticed. He didn't move around much during the day, but at night, when I was lying with my feet up, that's when he'd get all wriggly and start kicking me. Only he hadn't been kicking much in the last two weeks.'

'You can't blame yourself,' I said.

'When did it happen?' she asked. 'I'd just like to know. And why? I'm eight and a half months pregnant. Why did he come this far only to die now?'

She collapsed into tears, and that's when I took her in my arms and hugged her. It's all I could think to do, and in that moment it was the only comfort I had to offer. Tears formed in my own eyes. She was in such torment, stricken by grief, pain, confusion and guilt all at once. I couldn't begin to understand what she was going through. All I knew was that Jessica needed someone to hold her and tell her it wasn't her fault.

After an hour, I suggested she try to get some sleep. The labour was progressing well but she would need all her strength when it came to the actual birth. The only problem was that she was on antibiotics – she had a raised temperature when she came in, the first sign of an infection, so she was immediately put on antibiotics as a precaution. I had to go in every hour to administer these through her cannula.

Jessica had been dozing lightly on the bed, as I gently opened the door at midnight.

'Oh, here she is again!' Adam scoffed, rolling his eyes as I tiptoed into the room. He was a nice man, trying his best to lighten the mood at a dark time. 'You just can't keep away,' he added. 'She only dropped off five minutes ago.'

'Did I wake you? I'm so sorry, Jessica,' I said, 'but I've got to give you the antibiotics.'

'No, it's alright,' she sighed. 'I'm not sleeping really. Just dozing.'

Gradually, over the course of the night, I found out more and more about Jessica and Adam, and a strong bond formed between us. It was probably the worst night of their lives – the least I could do was be there for them both. We talked into the early hours about their lives, their hopes and aspirations.

Later, Jessica whispered into the darkness: 'Can I ask you something?' Adam was asleep on the armchair next to her bed. I was taking her observations.

'Of course.'

'What will he look like? I mean, will he look *normal*?'

Even though I'd not attended the birth of a stillborn before, I had seen a fair number of stillborn babies on the ward, so I did my best to reassure her.

'Yes, he'll be normal. He'll still be your baby. He was fine in all the scans, wasn't he? He looked fine then, so he's going to look fine when he's born. He'll still be warm; eventually, he will get cold, but you can hold him and spend as much time with him as you want. There'll be nothing wrong. The only difference will be that he's not alive.'

'Oh, I'm not sure about holding him.' Jessica sounded worried.

'Well, you don't have to make any decisions now,' I said. 'Just see how you feel when the time comes.'

She feared seeing what her child would look like. It was natural, after all, to be frightened of the unknown and I too felt trepidation, but I knew in my heart that he would be a normal baby.

At four in the morning, Jessica's pain changed, and she started to feel pressure and a pushing sensation. At that point Beverley came into the room and I stepped back a little. This was my first time, after all, and Beverley had the experience. I watched her deliver Jessica's boy, because I'd never seen anything like this before, and I'll admit I was apprehensive. But the baby came out quite quickly, which was a blessing. And he was beautiful. From his tiny eyes to his softly puckered mouth, he was perfect, just like a sleeping baby. The umbilical cord came out after him and that's when we saw the knot.

'It's a true knot,' Beverley said quietly. 'That was what happened to your son. While he was moving around inside the womb the cord knotted and pulled tight, cutting off his blood supply. There was nothing you or anyone could have done. I know it's no comfort right now, but it couldn't be helped.'

Beverley handed the boy to me and, in that moment, all my fears melted away. I noticed he was limp and felt heavier than a living baby. There was no tone to his limbs, and his eyes were closed. But apart from that, he was perfect. Another beautiful baby. I held their son for a little while as Jessica and Adam wept together. I cried, too. For the poor child I held in my arms and the parents who loved him. Together we grieved. Then I gave Jessica her son and, tentatively, slowly, she took him into her embrace.

'Oh, he's so lovely!' she exclaimed quietly in wonder. 'Look, Ads. Look how perfect he is.'

Adam couldn't speak. I guessed, in that moment, there were a million things going through his mind. A million possibilities for the boy he would have grown into, the man he would have become and the happiness he would have brought. And now, the gut-wrenching sadness he was feeling for this beautiful lifeless child in his wife's arms.

They named him Thomas, and for three days after the birth Jessica stayed in hospital, spending as much time with him as she could. It meant a lot to her to know the cause of his death, and to know that it was just bad luck, and nothing could have prevented it. Perhaps that knowledge made it slightly easier for her to accept. We looked after them throughout this time. We bathed him together and dressed him. We made a memory book with his tiny handprints and footprints and put in a lock of his hair, as well as dozens of photos. They also kept the baby label, which was on his ankles, a weight and length card confirming his date and time of birth, as well as a copy of the blessing book from the hospital chaplain. We talked to Jessica when she reached out to us but left her alone with Thomas when she seemed to want to share special time with him. And although it was horribly sad, there was something peaceful about allowing this grieving mother the time and space to mourn her child.

After three days, she didn't want to leave.

'I know I've got to, but I don't want to go,' she confided in me. I could understand – here, on this ward, Thomas was real. A real baby, a real presence whom she could hold and touch any time she liked. Going home meant leaving him behind, finally breaking that bond she had shared with her little boy for nearly nine months. Going home meant planning a funeral. Going home meant having to walk into the freshly painted nursery and seeing his little clothes all neatly folded, his cot for ever empty. Going home was the final twist of the knife in the loss of their baby.

A few weeks later, I came onto the ward at the start of my shift to see the whole reception desk and surrounding area covered in wine, chocolates, flowers and sweets.

'What's this all about?' I laughed. 'Are we opening a gift shop?'

'It was Adam,' replied Jen, the Labour Ward Coordinator. 'You remember the family that had a stillborn you looked after? The father brought all this lot in. Look, there's names on most of the presents and you've got a quite a few.'

I couldn't believe the generosity. Adam had bought us all gifts, each individually labelled. There were a few bottles of wine as well as a massive box of chocolates and some beautiful flowers for me. The gift-tag message was simple but heartfelt: 'We're so grateful for everything you did for us. Love, Jess, Adam and Thomas.'

As well as individual gifts, there were general gifts for the ward – many boxes of biscuits and giant tubs of sweets. It was completely over the top, but it made me feel so good. Because although they had suffered a devastating loss, the experience had been a positive one, and they were clearly happy with the care they'd received. I asked my manager if I could call them. It wasn't usually allowed but on this occasion she made an exception.

'You really didn't have to do that, but thank you for all your positive feedback. It means a lot to me,' I said.

* * *

Over the following years, Jessica and Adam kept up their connection to our ward. They did a lot of fundraising for improvements to the bereavement care suite and, I'm pleased so say, they returned two years later to give birth again – this time to a beautiful healthy little boy. I wasn't on shift when she delivered her baby but, thankfully, I was able to care for her after the birth and give her lots of breastfeeding support. It felt meaningful to us both. I didn't realise she'd had another one until I met her partner one day in Tesco, a couple of years later.

'It's Adam, isn't it?' I exclaimed when I saw him. He half-recognised me, so I explained that I'd helped deliver Thomas.

'And who is this?' I pointed to the tiny infant strapped up in the baby seat of his trolley.

'This is Henry,' he said, smiling. 'Our new baby!'

'Another boy?' I laughed.

'Yeah, another boy!'

* * *

In our third year of training, we all took on more respon-sibilities, both on the ward as well as in our community placements. It was a large teaching hospital and we would attend all the community antenatal clinics in the morning and then, in the afternoon, we'd go with the midwife to visit the women on their caseloads who had given birth, making sure they were okay. In the third year we also attended home births, usually as the second midwife, although on one occasion I was called out for a home birth as the main midwife.

At first, things didn't go according to plan. To begin with, I couldn't even find the house. It was on a new-build estate and my sat nav hadn't been updated, which meant it didn't recognise any of the roads. It just looked like I was driving around in a great big open space. I abandoned my car and started walking, asking anybody I could find if they knew where this road was. I eventually located the right cul-de-sac and was welcomed into the couple's lovely new town house by a bearded hulk of a man called Graham. He showed me into the lounge, where the French doors let in all the light from the garden, and in the middle of the floor was a fairly small and shallow birthing pool , in which his partner Nicky was sitting.

'Oh, you're here. Thank God!' she puffed. 'Find us alright, did you?'

'Yeah, fine,' I lied. I didn't want to give the wrong impression.

I did a quick check on Nicky, and found she was already quite advanced in labour, getting the occasional urge to push. But she seemed happy enough, and was coping well in the pool, so we agreed she should stay in there as long as she wanted. Just to be on the safe side, every fifteen minutes, I'd get her to stand up so I could listen to the baby's heartbeat, to make sure her baby was okay. In the meantime, I kept a close eye on the pool temperature and chatted to Graham, who seemed very relaxed about the imminent arrival of his first child.

'She knew she wanted to give birth at home,' he said, grinning. 'I mean, we moved in three weeks ago, brand-new carpets everywhere, and she wants a bloody pool birth!'

The first hour went smoothly but, after that, I had the Sonicade balanced on the side of the pool, while I counted the beats on my watch, and I must have been a little distracted because, a second later, the Sonicade wobbled and then toppled into the water.

Oh no! It's not waterproof!

I quickly fished it out and, just as I'd feared, the screen was completely blank. I shook it a couple of times before asking Graham whether he might have a couple of AA batteries. He took some out of the back of their TV remote control, but it was no good, the thing was kaput.

'I should have another one in here,' I said. I searched my midwife bag but the only thing I could find was a very old-fashioned pinard, which is like a metal horn for listening to the baby's heartbeat. There's a circle at one end, where you put your ear, and the wide end of the circle, at the other end, is placed on the abdomen. But you need utter silence to be able to hear the foetal heartbeat, and it wasn't really designed to be used in a pool birth. I was half-drowning trying to hear the baby's heartbeat! So, I called up my community midwife and asked her to come and assist, and to bring with her a new Sonicade.

'I think you better come now, Margaret,' I said. 'This lady's getting on in her labour.'

Of course, to Nicky and Graham, I didn't let on that there was anything amiss. They must have thought it was perfectly normal for a student midwife to keep dipping her head into the pool, getting half-soaked in the process, but there really was no other way with the pinard. The trouble was, Margaret didn't have a second Sonicade, and had to go all the way back to hospital to get one. Then, like me, she couldn't find the right road.

Time was ticking by. Meanwhile, Nicky was pushing. There was no getting away from the fact that this baby, a little girl, was on its way out. I had to do my best without the right kit – or a second midwife for that matter! *No need to panic,* I kept telling myself. *Everything's fine . . .*

On the surface, I was all smiles and encouragement, giving Nicky and Graham the impression that everything was under control. But inside, I was a real hot mess! I hadn't listened to the baby at all in the past hour because the Sonicade had broken. And the last hour of labour is the most stressful time for the baby, because that's when the head is being compressed and squashed.

Will she be okay? What should I do? Ring an ambulance and get her into hospital? No sign of Margaret! I'm just going to have to wing it . . .

'That's right,' I said, grinning at Nicky. 'You're doing really well. I can see the head. Now, another big push!'

By the time Margaret arrived, brandishing a new Sonicade, it was too late.

'She's coming!' I yelled. And at that moment, the baby slid out and into the pool and I scooped her up. She was in brilliant condition, which was such a relief because I had no way of knowing what was happening to her. Some people

47

worry about pool births because they think the newborn could drown, but they don't, because there are no pressure changes on the baby. The baby is already in water in the womb, so if they travel from water into water, they don't take their first gasp until they're lifted out. You just fish them out – their little nose twitches, their mouth opens, and they gasp, filling their tiny lungs with air for the first time.

The little girl gave her very first hiccupy cry. Nicky was ecstatic. The birth was just what she wanted – quiet, homely and intimate. She got out, wrapped a towelling robe round herself, and sat on her new sofa, cradling her newborn infant and grinning from ear to ear. Then she nodded to Graham: 'Right, tea and bacon rolls, I think. Yeah?'

Graham made us all a brew and bacon rolls, and we sat in that beautiful lounge while the late-afternoon sunlight streamed through the large windows, as Nicky breastfed her baby, dropping crumbs all over her perfect little head. It was lovely.

* * *

Of course, things can and do go wrong. You have to be prepared for that in childbirth, and I have to admit, even though I was quite good at staying calm in emergencies, there were times I felt like a rabbit in the headlights. For one birth in my final year, I was given a lovely lady called Tess to look after. It was a low-risk first birth and she had been progressing normally on just gas and air for a few hours. But then, as she entered the transitional stage, the pain started to get to her, tiring her out. She begged for some more pain relief and, although she was dead against having an epidural, she was happy to have a diamorphine injection. After I gave her the pain relief, she relaxed, and I let her doze for a bit before it was time to move her into the delivery room. Tess lay on the bed, eyes closed, asleep, I thought, mumbling a little incoherently. We wheeled her through the double doors into the delivery room, but now she needed to climb off the trolley and onto the bed herself, so I said: 'Come on, Tess, wake up. Let's get you onto this bed.'

Nothing. So I tried again.

'Hello? Come on, wake up. Wakey wakey! Come on, Tess, let's get you over. Tess? TESS?'

Nothing. She was totally unresponsive.

Now her partner tried to wake her – he was shaking her shoulder and practically shouting in her ear, but she was out for the count. I started to panic, and quickly checked her over: her blood pressure, heart, airways, all her observations were fine, which was strange. Diamorphine was a respiratory suppressant, so if she had reacted to the drug, you would think it would affect her breathing, but everything seemed normal. Except we couldn't wake her up. That definitely was *not* normal, because labouring women don't sleep deeply – it just isn't possible when your body is forcing out something the size of a watermelon through an extremely sensitive opening the size of a lemon. That tends to wake you up pretty sharpish! This lady clearly wasn't sleeping; she was unconscious.

I walked out of the room in a daze and announced to the people in the corridor: 'I think this lady's fallen unconscious in here.'

What was I thinking! I should have pulled the emergency buzzer. That's what it was there for. But I was so busy trying to stay calm and not overreact that I failed to do the one thing that would have alerted the team in the right way. In my confusion with the observations, I wasn't completely sure I had an emergency on my hands. Thankfully, my little announcement to the ward had the right effect.

'Unconscious?' said the midwife on the desk.

'Yeah,' I replied. 'I . . . er . . . I think she's reacted to the diamorphine.'

The whole team sprang into action. They quickly administered Narcan, a drug that reverses the diamorphine, and that brought her round very quickly. Tess woke up straight away and looked around her, almost like the scene in the movie *Pulp Fiction*, where Uma Thurman gets a shot of adrenaline and is startled by all the people in the room. We moved her onto a different bed but now, since the diamorphine effect had been reversed by the Narcan, she wasn't getting any pain relief and, as she was still contracting, she was in agony. We tried to tell her what had happened, but she was beside herself. 'Oh my God, is the baby alright? Is it alright?' she asked anxiously.

With reassurance she calmed back down, and as the diamorphine was no longer effective, due to having Narcan, she asked for an epidural.

In the end, Tess had a straightforward vaginal birth and everything was fine from that point on, but I was so shaken by the experience that I went to see her a lot after the birth, to make sure she was okay. I felt guilty and responsible – after all, I had given her the injection – and, for a while, it knocked my confidence. But Bev said I wasn't to let it affect me: 'You learn from your mistakes; you take things on board and move on.'

In the debrief, we talked about what we could have done differently and, in that instance, they said, 'Next time, just pull the emergency buzzer instead of coming out of the room.' *Doh!*

Funnily enough, I saw Tess not long afterwards, in Asda. It was lovely to bump into her again and she seemed really well.

'Oh my God, how are you? How's the baby?' I gushed. We chatted for a while, and then agreed to meet for coffee. We just seemed to click and, from there, we met for nights out at the pub together, went around each other's houses and, well, we've been friends ever since! When she fell pregnant again, I agreed to give her personal care for her second child.

She called me at 9 a.m. one morning, just as I was packing the last of my bags in the car.

'Pippa, I'm going into labour!' she puffed.

'Tess, I'm going to Center Parcs!' I replied.

Oh well. Plans change. We delayed our trip to Center Parcs for a few hours while I helped Tess through her second birth, and it was great. We had a special codeword, which meant the pain was too much and she wanted an epidural. So, when she said, 'Noodles', I knew she was serious. She delivered within five minutes of the anaesthetic taking effect. 'You didn't need it,' I tell her all the time. Tess is now thirty-five, and two years ago she started a midwifery course. 'You inspired me,' she said. 'I want to do what you do.' It is the greatest compliment anyone has ever paid me. Tess is now in her final year and will qualify in September and, in all honesty, I can't think of a better person to join our profession.

* * *

The Secret Midwife

By the end of my third and final year of training, our group of twenty had shrunk to thirteen. It shows just how tough the course was that so many of us had failed to make it to the end. I had been the youngest, and though I'd had my fair share of shocks and wobbles, I'd pushed myself hard to get to the finish line. The first day I pulled on my royal-blue dress, wrapped my belt around me and fastened my ornate silver buckle, I was filled with pride. Looking at myself in the mirror, I saw a different person to the immature, wide-eyed teenager who had started the course. I was confident, tougher, more assertive, and, though I doubted myself at times, I now had the resources and training to cope with practically anything. Thanks to a brilliantly supportive mentor and my amazing family – who never let me give up – I had found my feet. I was a midwife! Of course, you don't see everything in three years. There are some situations that no amount of training can prepare you for . . .

4

Expect the Unexpected

'Got a nice one for you, Pippa,' said Laura, the LWC, during handover. 'Low-risk second birth. Mum came in two hours ago, seems to be progressing well.'

It was the first week after I had qualified, and I was grateful to Laura to be given a low-risk, run-of-the-mill labour. Amanda was already 4 cms dilated when I took over her care in the low-risk birthing unit. There we had minimal medical equipment, fairy lights, scented aromatherapy candles, lots of cushions, couches and armchairs. It was a nice atmosphere. Her partner, Kane, was there, while Amanda's mother was at home with her four-year-old daughter. Amanda seemed to be coping well with the pain. She'd had a spontaneous vaginal birth the first time around, so we were expecting the same again.

'I hear the second often comes quicker than the first. Gotta be ready!' Kane joked.

'That does happen a lot,' I agreed. 'I've had some ladies deliver their second or third baby within minutes.'

'Do you catch them every time?'

'*Most* of the time,' I said, smiling in response.

Things moved along at a fair pace and the atmosphere in the room was jolly and upbeat. Amanda coped with just gas and air, and within the hour she was fully dilated and feeling the urge to push, so she started to bear down. I wasn't taking any chances: I was all set with my tray, ready to catch. But the minutes ticked past and no baby – it seemed no matter how hard Amanda pushed, this baby wasn't coming. I tried bending down to get a look, and though I could just about see the crown, it wasn't moving. There was no descent. Amanda was trying really hard, but nothing was happening. *Why isn't this baby coming?* I wondered. *Maybe we need to change her position?*

We moved her to a high-dependency room where we had more equipment and put her on the monitor to get a scan of her baby's heartbeat. At this stage, we would normally expect a nice steady line, but I wasn't happy with the CTG scan at all. Amanda's baby was showing accelerations – which is where the line goes up – and decelerations, where the line dips below that baseline. The decelerations indicated that the baby's heart rate was slowing during Amanda's contractions. It was recovering back up again afterwards, but the decelerations worried me. It appeared the baby was in distress and something needed to be done.

'I'm going to get the doctor to come in and review you,' I told Amanda.

I called in the registrar. In any hospital ward, there are different kinds of doctors and it can get a little confusing if you don't know the jargon but, just to explain . . . back in the days before the 'modernising medical careers', different titles indicated the different levels of skill and expertise. The structure went like this: on the first rung of the ladder was the Senior House Officer (or SHO), who is a junior doctor; the registrar (or Reg) was higher in seniority, and then, above them all, was the consultant. Since the consultant is very senior, he does ward rounds in the morning and is then often in consultation or surgery in the afternoon. At night, the consultant is 'on call', meaning they are not necessarily in the hospital but are available to attend in the case of a very serious emergency. These days all the titles have changed, so you're no longer an SHO but an F2. It's seriously confusing, so we all still think in terms of the old classifications.

The registrar examining Amanda decided to carry out an assisted delivery with a ventouse suction cup. The cup was carefully applied to the baby's head and he attempted to pull the baby out, but it failed. He then opted for a forceps delivery. Forceps are like a pair of giant salad tongs, which the doctor uses to grab hold of the baby's head to pull it out. The registrar took hold of the tongs and gave a good pull. Then he tried again – the rule is: three pulls maximum. So he tried one last time, in hope, but this baby wasn't budging.

'Okay, Amanda, we're going to take you into theatre now, because we might have to do a caesarean to get your baby out safely,' I told her, while Kane was taken away to be given a pair of scrubs and gloves. It was important to keep talking to them both, to let them know what was going on.

'Is he okay?' Amanda asked anxiously, as I held her hand. 'Is the baby okay?'

'Yes, he's fine, but we need to get him out fairly soon, and we need to ensure it'll be the safest way for both of you.'

She nodded, putting her full trust in us all, and I felt

that responsibility keenly. Now she was wheeled straight into theatre, and the decision to call in the consultant was made. At this point Amanda was still fully conscious but she hadn't had much pain relief, so we gave her a spinal once she was in theatre, which numbed her from the bust down. When the consultant arrived, we all felt a shared sense of relief – it was Professor Andrews, the head of department. The Prof had the mantra of 'If I do it, so can you' with his surgical team, so he was never one to shun on-call rotas or push them to more junior consultants. He was one of a rare breed. All the staff and patients loved him.

The Prof introduced himself to Amanda and Kane and, once pleasantries were over, he examined her and decided to attempt a forceps delivery one last time before surgery – just the one pull, however, as the registrar had already attempted forceps. Using forceps means applying a fair amount of pressure to a baby's head, which is not damaging in the long term but can result in some serious cuts and bruising. The forceps failed again, so the only remaining option was to carry out an emergency C-section. So far, so normal. Most caesarean sections are planned in advance, but emergency C-sections happen all the time, and for various different reasons. Quite often, if the baby is breech or in an awkward position, it can make a vaginal delivery very difficult, but the doctors try their best to avoid surgery by attempting to get the baby out with suction or forceps. It's all a question of urgency. If the baby needs to come out straight away, we'll move directly to surgery, but as this carries risks, it is usually the last resort.

Since we'd prepared Amanda and her partner by telling them what was happening, they both accepted the Prof's decision readily. As far as they were concerned, the only thing that mattered was getting their baby out safely. They trusted us completely and they had good reason to. After all, they now had every doctor on the ward in theatre with them: the Prof, the registrar and SHO, as well as a whole specialist team. The Prof began his incision and, within minutes, out came Amanda's little boy, safe and sound. As soon as Professor Andrews lifted him up, I could see what the problem had been – he was gigantic! A very large baby weighing in at 10 lbs 2 ounces. That was the reason he hadn't been able to descend through the birth canal. He had a couple of cuts and bruises, but nothing abnormal for a forceps delivery, and the happy parents were relieved that their son was okay.

The section complete, Professor Andrews now left the theatre while the registrar and SHO were tasked with suturing the section site then swabbing the remaining blood from out through the vagina. In other words, sewing and cleaning her up. Meanwhile, I took charge of their little boy. I was just conducting the last of the checks when Amanda started to bleed heavily. And I mean *heavily*. It was like somebody had turned on a tap. Everyone's eyes in theatre widened in shock as it poured out of her, cascading off the bed and onto the floor, turning everything in its path a crimson red. The team leaped into action, but you could sense the panic in the air as the registrar tried to cope with the sheer quantity of blood gushing out of Amanda.

Where was it coming from? How could he stop it? If a woman bled after a C-section, it was usually from the uterus, but all the usual techniques to stop the flow didn't seem to be working. The registrar and SHO now spoke to one another in quiet but urgent tones, back and forth:

SHO: 'I think perhaps we should call back the Prof.'

Reg: 'I don't need you to *think*, I need you to help me find what's haemorrhaging and clamp it.'

SHO: 'I can't see anything, it's flooding.'

Reg (turning back to the anaesthetist): 'Can we get more clotting drugs administered?'

SHO: ' I just can't see . . . it's a fucking flood!'

Reg: 'I need more suction, please, more suction and we should see it, get ready to clamp.'

SHO: 'Clamp what? There is nothing to clamp! We *need* the Prof back!'

Reg: 'We can handle this – it's just a bleed. I NEED MORE SUCTION! Nurse, can we double-check the placenta is complete?'

It was 7 p.m. and I was due to finish my shift and go into handover to let the next shift come on, but I couldn't just walk away and leave Amanda like this. The registrar had undone the sutures in order to get a look at what was happening, but they hadn't yet located the cause of the bleeding. By now Amanda's partner had been taken out of the room with the baby. Amanda, meanwhile, had been put under with a general anaesthetic when she started to bleed. I stood there, poised to leave, but before I did, I spoke up.

'Shall I get help?' I asked the registrar.

'We're fine at the minute,' he muttered, without looking up. 'We'll deal with this.'

It didn't *look* fine, and it didn't *seem* like he was dealing with it. I took a step back towards the door and saw the scene as if in slow motion: Amanda lying there, stomach cut wide open, the sheets and surgeons both drenched red.

The only thing they were dealing with right now was the possibility of leaving a baby without a mum.

Right, I thought. *I don't care what he says – he needs help.* If it was this man's pride versus this woman's life, there was no competition. I walked out of theatre and straight to the phone. I rang the switchboard, cleared my throat, then spoke loudly and clearly: 'We need help in theatre four. Can you please call the obstetric consultant, Professor Andrews?'

It didn't matter that I was the most junior midwife in the hospital, just a week qualified; it didn't matter that I was shaking, thinking I was going to get the sack for going above a doctor's instructions. What did matter was Amanda needed help and she needed it straight away. Anyone could see that! I knew in my heart that no matter the repercussions for my actions, my conscience would be clear. Then I headed back into theatre to assist.

Amanda was already six litres of blood down when the consultant burst through the doors. 'Why wasn't I called immediately?' he roared. By now she had been hooked up to a blood transfusion, but they couldn't get it into her quick enough before it was coming out again. Everyone was starting to get nervous. There was a real danger that if we couldn't stop the blood flow, Amanda would bleed out. Professor Andrews's brow furrowed in concentration as he worked swiftly, trying to figure out where the bleeding was coming from so he could stop the flow. He had tried inserting another Bakri Balloon, which is like a large bag that you can inflate inside the uterus to stop bleeding, but that had made no difference. He was running out of options to save this woman's life.

Eventually, he looked at his surgical team and gave the

sharp words: 'I'm going to remove everything. Anyone here have any objections?' The room fell silent apart from the rhythmic beeps and low whine of the machines supplying life. I didn't fully understand what he meant, but it didn't take long to find out. The Prof asked for a new scalpel, then extended the already monstrous cut across Amanda's belly to about a foot wide. It looked like she had been sawn in half. He worked quickly with precision, still fighting through the crimson torrent that continued to fill and pour from her lifeless body. Once he'd completed the full hysterectomy, and was sure the bleeding had stopped, he sutured her internals, pulled himself bolt upright, took off his mask and sighed heavily. It was like everyone had been holding their breath until that moment, and now, finally, we could breathe normally again. The immediate danger had passed.

'Right, I'm going out for a smoke,' he said glumly. 'I'll come back to finish up.'

He went outside for a cigarette, came back in, put on fresh scrubs and gloves and carried on until Amanda was stable enough to be taken to ITU. By that point, she had been in theatre for nearly five hours.

I left the theatre in a daze but, the moment I got home, I started to shake. And then the tears overtook me. I couldn't believe how quickly the situation had changed. Everything was fine one minute, then the next we were facing a full-blown emergency. I lay on my bed and cried my eyes out that night, just letting the tears roll. I had stayed calm throughout the crisis but, as soon as I was home, all those natural reactions of shock and fear that I'd managed to keep under control rose to the surface. I'd been so very frightened she was going to die.

Expect the Unexpected

Amanda was in ITU for the next four days, and I went in every day to see her, to make sure she was recovering well. I was in a state of shock myself in the days after the crisis. My mind raced with worry and doubts started to creep in about my own actions and abilities.

Was it something I did? Or didn't do? Was I too complacent? Could I have prevented the situation developing into a crisis if I had done something different? What if I'd realised sooner that the baby was too big?

These questions preyed on my mind for weeks afterwards. But in the debrief Laura, the LWC, was full of praise. She congratulated me for having the presence of mind to alert the Prof and not feel threatened by the doctors when I thought something was wrong. That made me feel slightly better – at least I had the right instincts. Even if it had been a false alarm, she said, I had made the right judgement call, and after that I could sleep soundly, knowing I'd done everything I could to ensure Amanda's safety.

* * *

The more I worked in the job, the more I learned to trust my own instincts. And I learned how to read people, to see beyond their bravado, to tell when they were unsure and to act accordingly – because even when their mouths said one thing their behaviour might tell an entirely different story. Through experiences like this, I found my assertiveness and I became more and more confident as time went on. It didn't stop getting to me, though, and that was something I hadn't quite realised when I started out – the emotional cost. I had no idea just how much I would end up taking the job home with me.

The Secret Midwife

You can't go through those kinds of experiences and not be affected. Every couple of weeks there would be some new drama, and I'd come home and sob my heart out. I just needed to get it off my chest. Or there were times I came off a shift at the point where a lady was about to deliver and, instead of focusing on my own life, I'd obsess about that woman, ringing up the ward in the middle of the night to find out whether she had delivered safely.

It's not a nine-to-five job, that's for sure. The high of seeing a mum's face when she first sets eyes on her child is unbeatable. That's the best bit of my job, handing mum her baby and looking at their faces, both of them together, as they see each other for the first time. What an honour to be there, sharing that special moment! But childbirth is a dangerous business, and the lows are there too. You learn to roll with the punches. You learn to take the bitter with the better.

5

Mother Knows Best?

I got used to a lot of different aspects of the job fairly quickly. I became an expert photographer, managing to grab the camera at exactly the right moment to capture that magical first cuddle of the parents with their newborn child. I became adept at avoiding getting pinched or grabbed by women in pain, although my methods weren't always foolproof, and I even got bitten once. I can't say I was all that impressed.

'Ow! Bite your husband!' I ordered. 'Then we can send him to A&E.'

And I got used to answering a million questions from anxious parents who had scoured the internet and managed to find the most obscure complications they felt certain applied to them. I didn't mind; it was all part of the job. Especially the answering questions part – it was normal to worry, and now, thanks to the internet, we all had a thousand more reasons to feel anxious. And although I was usually happy to be challenged on what I was doing, it wasn't always appropriate. In fact, there was one occasion in my early years of midwifery when the mother really did think she knew best – and it tested me to my very limits.

Diana had come in fairly soon after her waters broke, and from the word go I had concerns. The waters were thick and green with meconium, and almost the consistency of pea soup. It meant the baby had pooed a lot in her waters, and that was not a good sign. Babies usually only poo into the amniotic sac when they are under stress. If that baby then took the meconium into its lungs, it could cause an infection. The first thing we needed to do was find out how the baby was coping, and for that I needed to monitor the heartbeat. But Diana had other ideas.

'I don't want anybody listening to my baby's heartbeat,' she said firmly. 'I just want to do this on my own, without outside interference.'

'But I just need to check your baby is okay,' I countered. 'Your waters indicate your baby could be in distress. I just want to listen in to your baby.'

'No.'

'But your baby, at the minute, is at risk of infection. I really would like to listen in to your baby.'

'No. I can feel my baby. My baby's fine.'

Diana's husband Mike was by her side, biting hard on his nails. By the look of his fingers, he'd been doing this a lot recently.

He remained silent the whole time. Then, as I was preparing the room, he whispered quietly to his wife: 'Di, don't you think we should just let them listen?'

'NO!' she shouted back, with such force it made me jump. 'I told you, if you can't support my decisions then you're not welcome in here. We agreed, remember? We agreed to do this naturally.'

'Yup, yup, that's right.' Mike shrank back into his plastic chair. 'But if the midwife here says it's safer, then . . .'

'I don't want the monitor, okay? So just drop it,' Diana snapped.

Hmm . . . I'll have to try another tack.

Over the next hour, I pulled in every single senior member of the team I could find on the ward. Laura, the LWC, had a go at talking Diana round. Next, it was the turn of the senior house officer, then I cornered the registrar, and he tried his best to convince her into letting us put her on the monitor and, finally, I pulled out my secret weapon: Angela. If silver-tongued Angela couldn't talk this lady round, I don't know who could.

'So, you see, my darling,' Angela explained, 'you're doing so well, but your little one could be in trouble in there and we need to help them out. We know it's not your first choice, but safety first, hmmmm?'

'I'll tell you what I told all those others,' Diana huffed. 'I don't want the monitor. I don't want any interference. If I say my baby is okay, it's okay. Now why do I keep getting harassed like this?'

'Alright, my dear, alright. I hear you,' Angela soothed, then threw me a look before she crept out of the room. *What now? I was at my wits' end!*

'I can't do it,' I told Laura twenty minutes later. 'I can't look after that woman any more. I can't be responsible for her baby. It's too serious. If that child dies it will be on my shoulders, but she's not letting me do anything to help!'

'You've got to keep at it, Pippa,' Laura said. 'Whatever

happens we're noting everything down, so it'll be on record that you have tried to use the monitor.'

'Tried? I have *battled* with that woman for hours! She is just so stubborn. I just don't know where she's getting this idea from that she knows better than we do. We're the ones with the medical expertise and we're telling her that her baby is at risk. What right has she got to put her baby in harm's way like this? It's so selfish . . . and cruel!'

By now, I was fuming, and I swiped at angry tears.

'You are doing a brilliant job, Pippa,' said Laura, putting a comforting hand on my shoulder. 'But you can't force her to have monitoring. She has to be accountable for her own actions. You can only try to persuade her. I know you can do it. Take a minute, compose yourself and get back in there. I get it. I really do. But we all have to go through these things. Just do your best.'

So I did. I supported Diana while she contracted and, just like with the monitor, she declined any pain relief.

'*Nnnnn . . . aaaaughhhhh!*' she screamed, as the contractions started to pick up in speed and intensity. It wasn't a 'good scream', not at all. The next contraction, I was just bending down, about to put a towel compress on her back, when I felt her hand grab my neck and her long fingernails dug deep into my skin.

'*Argh!*' Now it was my turn to scream. I put my hand up to my neck. *Blood!* She'd dug her long talons into my neck so hard she'd drawn blood.

'That is not necessary, Diana,' I said crossly. 'We have pain relief for that.'

'Oh, sorry, sorry, sorry,' she panted. 'I didn't know it was you.'

'Just keep your hands to yourself, please!' I added pointedly.

The hours rolled on and still Diana refused to let us take any heart readings from her baby. I couldn't understand how a normal person, with no medical background or training, thought she knew better than a whole ward full of experts. It was baffling. She didn't seem like any kind of 'Earth Mother' type; there was nothing particularly hippyish about her. She was just extraordinarily stubborn.

She maintained that since it was *her* body she knew better than anyone else what she was going through. Her partner Mike didn't say much. I guessed if he'd had his way we would have been able to put her on the monitor straight away, but then Diana was a very domineering character. Even though she was fairly small in stature, she was fierce, and she overpowered him completely. But I didn't give up – just like Laura said, I kept up the pressure because I knew it was the only way to help Diana's baby. And, finally, through a combination of her tiredness from the contractions and my persuasion, I wore her down. Four hours after she came onto the ward she let me listen to her baby's heartbeat.

Oh my God. My body went cold when I saw the line on the monitor. I had never seen such a horrible trace in all my life. The heartbeat was all over the place, swinging high and low. This baby was in deep distress. I called in the registrar, Dr Pellitz, straightaway, and she too was alarmed by what she saw.

'Your baby is in distress,' she explained quietly and seriously to Diana and Mike. 'This can be very dangerous for a baby, and it can mean your baby is not getting enough oxygen. If we don't get your baby out quickly, lack of oxygen can lead to brain damage or even death, so I suggest that we go for an immediate delivery in theatre. We could try forceps, but if that doesn't work we would proceed to a caesarean.'

Since Diana hadn't let us examine her, we had no idea where she was in her labour, so we couldn't decide the best plan to deliver baby safely until we'd had a look. All we knew was that baby needed out, and fast!

'No. No way,' Diana panted. 'I'm not having any of that.'

'But we are very concerned about your baby.'

'No interventions. No!'

A long silence ensued, as Dr Pellitz turned away from Diana and directed her attention at Mike. He had hold of Diana's hand and was looking at his wife, refusing to meet Dr Pellitz's gaze, but she continued to stare questioningly at him, even as Diana yelled through another contraction.

'NO, MIKE. I SAID NO INTERVENTIONS!' she shouted. Eventually he sighed and shook his head.

'It's what she says.' He shrugged hopelessly. 'I can't make her.'

'Well, that is your choice as the parents,' Dr Pellitz replied. 'But it's my job to help deliver your baby safely, and if I can't do that then I must make you aware of the possible consequences. I'm sorry but this is very, very serious.'

I wanted to scream. I wanted to grab that stupid woman by the shoulders and give her a good shake. *We're trying to save your baby, you stupid idiot!* Her arrogance was breathtaking, but there was nothing we could do. It took another hour for Diana to push her baby out and, by the time the little girl was born, we had five members of the team ready on standby for resuscitation. Fortunately, the baby breathed from the moment she slid out, although she was pale and stained a greenish tinge due to the meconium.

When we took gas readings from the cord, we discovered she had very low PH levels. This indicated the baby had been oxygen deprived for quite some time and was suffering hypoxia. There was a high chance that she was permanently brain damaged.

'See! She's fine. She's fine!' Diana cried, as she put her arms out to hold her little girl.

'She's not fine,' the doctor said sternly. 'She is hypoxic and possibly brain damaged. We need to send her for cooling straight away to preserve brain activity.'

'But I don't want– ' Diana started to object.

'It's not your decision now,' Dr Pellitz cut in, her temper now at breaking point. 'It is now the decision of the neonatal intensive care and paediatric team. They have to, and will, do what is best for the interests of their patient. So, let me be very clear, whether you agree or disagree, your baby is being transferred for cooling in the very slim hope that we are able to salvage some brain activity.'

She promptly turned, thanked us all and walked out of the room, muttering under her breath.

I was coming to the end of my shift and I didn't stick around to hear any more. The baby was wheeled away and I left to write up the paperwork – which takes around two hours for each birth. I had given Diana the best possible care but I could barely look at her. The whole experience had stretched me to my very limits. If I spent any more time in that woman's company I couldn't account for what I would do to her. To my mind, she was 100 per cent responsible for damaging her own child.

I knew the heartbeat would be erratic just from seeing those thick, foul waters. And yet, when it was finally confirmed, she still wouldn't listen. If we had got that baby out within an hour or two of her arrival, that child would most likely be perfectly healthy. Instead, Diana and Mike were facing an uncertain future of caring for a brain-damaged child. I didn't feel sorry for them but for the poor innocent child they had harmed. The little girl was sent to another hospital that had the right equipment for advanced cooling, but I didn't have the heart to follow up. I couldn't bear to hear how their story ended because, to my mind, it could have all been so different.

The fact is, mothers don't always know best, and some mothers actively harm their children before they are even born. I got used to dealing with mothers in labour who had a history of either drinking or using drugs – or both. Most of them were honest and they'd tell you if they used. In most cases they couldn't hide it because they were already known to Social Services, and it was all there in their notes. If they were being monitored, we had access to their drug-test results that showed whether they had been using during pregnancy. But others wouldn't admit to it for fear of having their baby taken away from them. You can tell, though. Heavy drinking during pregnancy can lead to Foetal Alcohol Syndrome [FAS], which is clear to see from the moment a baby is born. Their eyes are further apart, and they usually have thin lips, a small head, and a smooth ridge between the upper lip and nose. They are also born with low birth weight. If we suspect they are suffering from FAS, we'll refer that family to Social Services straight away, but a lot of the time they are already known and under consultant care.

Cocaine use in pregnancy is on the rise, and of course this can often be damaging. It can cause the placenta to come away before the baby's born, depriving it of oxygen and blood supply. Not even marijuana is harmless. Some still do it, even when they're in labour. They'll go off ward and come back red-eyed and sleepy. We know they're stoned but they won't admit it. It can affect the baby's heart rate, making it speed up, a condition known as tachycardia. And for the harder drugs, well, there's nothing quite so heartbreaking as seeing a newborn baby withdrawing. There's certainly no mistaking their high-pitched, ear-piercing cries echoing down the corridors.

One twenty-three-year-old known heroin user had come in at thirty-one weeks with a complication in her pregnancy, and we had admitted her to the ward for observation. I was on the night shift, and, as I went around, seeing all the women, I noticed that Julie wasn't there.

'Where's Julie Lyons?' I asked my colleagues. Nobody had seen her and she didn't appear to be in any of the rooms. I was concerned – she was clearly a vulnerable individual and we had a responsibility to keep an eye out for her while she was in our care.

'Looks like she's absconded,' sighed Jen, the Labour Ward Coordinator on that night.

'What should we do?' I asked.

'Well, let's give her an hour or so, see if she turns up, and if she's not back by midnight, we'll call the emergency duty team to advise. We may have to inform the police.'

At 11.50 p.m., Julie walked back onto the ward – or rather, she crept back. I think she thought we wouldn't notice.

'Hi there, Julie!' I called down the corridor, as I noticed her trying to sneak back into her room without being seen.

'Oh, yeah, hi,' she drawled. 'Erm . . . wass yer name?'

'It's Pippa. Remember?'

'Hmmm?'

Julie had left the ward in a normal state but had returned completely out of it. Her eyes were glazed over, she walked and moved really slowly, and her speech was slurred.

'Where've you been, Julie?' I asked casually.

'Oh . . . out . . . jusss chatting to m' friends,' she said, her eyelids half closed.

'Have you taken anything, love?' I asked.

'Nope.' She shook her head slowly and swayed gently with the motion.

'Are you sure?'

'Yup. Jusss wanna take a bath. Is that okay?'

'Yeah, okay, Julie. I'll see you in a little while.'

I discussed the situation with Jen, who said we should keep an eye on her, so I let her have a bath while I attended a woman in the early stages of labour in another room. Then, at 12.15 a.m., I went to check on Julie, knocking on her bathroom door. No answer. I tried the handle. Locked! *Uh-oh. This isn't good.* I went to fetch Jen and she brought her master key – quickly, she got the door unlocked, and that's when we saw the carnage.

It was like a scene out of a Quentin Tarantino movie. Julie was passed out in the bath with only her nose above the water, which was a deep crimson colour. Cigarette butts floated in the water next to her limp body and a razor blade dangled loosely from her fingers on the outside of the bath.

Oh my God! What's going on? Is she dead?

For a moment, I tried to take it all in, and then I saw the cuts along her bump. She had been slashing at her belly with the blade in a bizarre attempt to give herself a DIY caesarean. Jen and I rushed forward together and, in one swift motion, we took an arm each, wrenching Julie clear of the water. I yanked the emergency cord and the whole team piled into the bathroom.

'Julie! Julie! Are you awake?' I shouted, as my colleague placed a towel over the cuts and compressed them to try to stop the bleeding. Meanwhile, Jen made sure she had clear airways and supported her head. A fourth midwife checked her observations and the fifth called the registrar. Once Julie started to come round, and was stable, we got her onto a resus bed and waited for the doctors. We worked quietly but swiftly to attend to the worst of her injuries. During those moments it's a question of putting on your poker face and trying to stay calm and composed. Even in the worst emergencies you work as a team, knowing that everyone who needs to be there is there. It's only later at home that you let yourself cry. We found out later that the cuts hadn't been deep enough to get below to the uterus, but it was a frightening experience and the doctors called for the Motherhood Mental Health Team to review her the following day on the ward, before transferring her to a mental health unit for professional support. Julie clearly had a troubled past and was struggling in her life. I hoped that she would now get the help she so desperately needed.

To this day, I don't know what possessed her to take such

dreadful actions, and I know that if she had been in her right mind she would never have done something like that, but there is no escaping the fact that sometimes we are called on to protect babies even from the mothers who are carrying them. It sounds crazy, doesn't it? Most of us can't imagine doing anything harmful to our children, and have an innate sense of protecting a baby or an unborn child. But there are exceptions to every rule. And whether it is from an irrational mind like Diana's, or a disturbed one like Julie's, I have learned from personal experience that mothers do not always know best.

6

Chameleons

We're like chameleons, us midwives, adapting our personalities to match the families we look after. If I walk into a birthing suite to find the mother is effing and blinding all over the place, I'm a little bit more relaxed with my own language and demeanour. But if the family are well-spoken, then I'm careful to keep my language clean and professional at all times. But there is one thing that never changes: I am the mother's advocate. I am there to ensure her needs and wishes are heard and that she feels informed and in control of what's happening to her. After all, this is her body, her birth, her child – and some mums have been planning this day for years. Of course, things change, and childbirth never quite goes according to plan, but it's important that we try to get every woman the experience she wants. After all, you only get one chance to get this right. I am that mother's voice, even when she is in too much pain to speak. And if that means fighting to get her an epidural, I'll get her that damn epidural! It's no secret that some anaesthetists can be a bit stubborn, however.

'What baby number is this?' they'll quiz me, when I dare to put in a request.

'How many centimetres is she? Is she going to deliver quickly?'

I wave away their questions. 'It doesn't matter. She needs an epidural. So please come and give her an epidural.'

'Well, she might have delivered by the time I get there.'

'That's true, and, if that's the case, brilliant. But then again, she might not have. So come on!'

I always deliver my requests with a smile, but the soft exterior is only there to hide the steely resolve inside. I won't be the one to back down.

For every woman that gives birth on our ward there are a different set of considerations and risks to weigh up, prompting a discussion with the whole team around their care. Pool births can often be a point of disagreement between midwives and doctors. For a woman to be able to go into a pool she must be low risk, with no complicating factors, and a good 4–5 cms dilated. But if they have risk factors – for example, a raised BMI, a large estimated foetal weight or a previous section – then the attending doctor may object. Depending on how the woman is managing, I might then try to persuade the doctor to allow them to have the experience they so deeply desire.

'Let's put her in for now and see how she gets on,' I'll suggest. 'After all, her pregnancy so far has been pretty low risk, her admission CTG is normal with good movements, and she is able to get in and out of the pool.'

I get my way quite often. It is a question of trust between

the professionals on the ward. The consultants and doctors respect our opinion as midwives – they know we're capable of looking after these women – so they will give us the benefit of the doubt. Even if a woman is only a couple of centimetres along and isn't ready to give birth, she might not want to go home, so I will use the pool to help calm and relax her. My mantra is – whatever works! If you want to sit on a birthing ball, lovely. If you want to walk up and down the corridor, great. If you would prefer to be in the pool, that works for us too.

It's all about careful monitoring. If we keep a close eye on our ladies, we know exactly how the birth is coming along. In my first couple of years as a midwife, I came across a fair few women who told me they wanted what is known in birthing jargon as a VBAC – a Vaginal Birth After a Caesarean section. I couldn't see a problem, but the doctors weren't always so keen. My feeling was that as long as there weren't any other risk factors, those women should at least have the option to try a vaginal birth.

'I just want to *try* to push this one out,' one woman told me. 'I failed the last time.'

'Failed? What do you mean?'

'I mean, I had to have a C-section and I really didn't want one.'

'Yes, but that doesn't mean you failed.'

'Oh, really!' she scoffed. I looked through the notes from her first baby and written over every page was that dreadful phrase, 'failed to progress'. My heart sank. I hate those words. I never use them myself, but it's still the most common shorthand by doctors and midwives to describe a labour that doesn't advance at the expected rate. I write:

'Did not pass further than 3 cms' or 'Did not dilate further than 4 cms'. Language is important. Women pick up on the words we use, and that experience stays with them throughout the pregnancy and labour, making them feel as if they are being judged.

Failed. It is so harsh, placing an unfair emphasis on the mother when the truth is, it is totally out of her control. Giving birth is a physical process, not a moral judgement. The language we use impacts on how mothers feel about themselves from the word go. And telling them they've 'failed' before they've even started seems to me so wrong. At the very least women should be told how frequent C-sections are.

At our hospital we do at least two elective (that means pre-arranged) sections a day, plus a handful of emergency C-sections. And that's not a high rate! At some of the busier hospitals there can be up to eight to ten every day. Having a caesarean section is not a sign of failure; it is purely a medical procedure to ensure the safe arrival of your baby. And whether that decision is made weeks in advance or on the day, it is the same thing. Words matter. For example, I never like to call my women 'patients'. Why would I? They're not sick – they're having a baby, which is a perfectly natural thing to do. I usually call the women I look after by their names or 'ladies', but I never use the term 'patient'.

Besides anything else, it is up to us, the experts, to do our best to keep things moving, but I sometimes find our own advice doesn't help with that. When women are put on the hormone drip, quite often the doctors will advise them to lie on the bed. But this is so restricting, and we know that lying down isn't always helpful in advancing labour. So we get them up and walking around, even if they're walking around with a drip in one hand.

Fortunately, I'm lucky enough to have landed at a hospital where the team works really well together and the midwives have a great relationship with the doctors. They trust our opinion and let us lead the way. We like to watch and observe and try different techniques before resorting to an assisted birth. It's not the same everywhere. In some hospitals there is a stronger doctor-led culture. They don't like to sit on things, so, if something is causing concern, they'll just get the baby out – consequently, there are higher C-section rates in some hospitals compared to others.

Of course, we follow the NICE guidelines (the National Institute for Health and Care Excellence, the body that sets all the clinical guidelines within the NHS), but the whole culture of birth management differs from one unit to the next. Even the make-up of your team on the day can affect the outcome – after all, each midwife is different, and each doctor has different judgement. Some doctors will insist on a hormone drip if they think the woman has been labouring too long on her own. Depending on the doctor, I might then be able to persuade them to give her a few more hours to allow her body to try and do it. Those few extra hours could be decisive in the birth she ends up having. It's about giving her time and not making her feel rushed.

As much as we consult and request attendance from our doctors, there are occasions when it is simply better if they stay away. During my first couple of years at one NHS Trust, I worked with a doctor who was notorious for her poor bedside manner. Dr Matthews didn't mean to be rude; it was just her way of communicating. One woman was unsure about having a diamorphine injection and couldn't make up her mind whether she needed the pain relief or not. At which point, Dr Matthews exploded: 'Well, am I doing this, or shall I just walk back out again? It's your choice.'

The woman just stared at her, nonplussed, uncertain how to respond to this ultimatum. And then Dr Matthews walked out.

'I'm so sorry about that,' I started to apologise.

'Is she normally like that or is it just me?'

'Oh no, don't worry. She's like that with everyone.'

And yet, there's just no excuse for that kind of behaviour. Ten minutes later, Dr Matthews reappeared at the door.

'Are you ready for me yet?' she barked. At that, the woman and I exchanged a look and we both burst out laughing.

'How do you put up with her?' she asked, after Dr Matthews left.

'It really helps to have a sense of humour,' I replied. Thank goodness she hadn't got upset.

I couldn't always see the funny side of Dr Matthews's abrupt manner, though. There was one occasion I watched her order a woman around during a forceps delivery, and it was horrible and humiliating.

'Put your legs up,' she barked at the poor woman. 'No! Not like that. Like this. Arm over here, just like this . . . no, that's not right.' She was treating her worse than an animal.

'Ahem,' I cleared my throat. 'Can we do one thing at a time, *please*, Doctor?'

Dr Matthews didn't like that, but she got my point, and after my interruption, she slowed down and added the odd 'please' and 'thank you'. But generally, she didn't much bother with politeness or social niceties. I think in her opinion the medical aspect was all that mattered, and social skills weren't necessary. But I learned how to deal with Dr Matthews, too, keeping my tone firm but light-hearted in order to get my point across without sounding aggressive.

One lady found Dr Matthews so offensive that she ordered me to 'keep that bitch away'. So I had to ensure that she never came into her room. It wasn't easy. This particular mother-to-be was pushing for quite some time and Dr Matthews kept hanging around outside.

'Do you need any help?' she called out from behind the door every half an hour or so. 'Does she need a lift out?'

'No, thanks. We're fine.'

'Can I come in?'

'No, sorry. This room is closed.'

'You need to keep me updated,' she huffed.

'Everything's fine. Trust me!' I called out pleasantly. 'We'll let you know if they are any problems.'

We all muddled along, but after a couple of years Dr Matthews found a better position in another hospital, and I can't say I was terribly disappointed when she announced her departure. She was a good doctor, but when you're dealing with people at such a sensitive time, I believe you have to employ a whole range of skills to get the best outcome.

* * *

Different people want different things, and sometimes there are cultural considerations to take on board. The Travelling community are one such group who often have a completely different set of norms and expectations when it comes to giving birth. To begin with, no matter how much they travel or where they go, many will prefer to return to the same hospital every time to give birth. I noticed this early on, when I started to recognise the names as they came up on our ward over and over again.

'Rosie Malley, is it? I recognise you. Didn't you give birth here three years ago?' I asked one lady.

'Oh yes,' Rosie replied proudly. 'I have all my babies here.'

They like things a certain way. All the female relatives accompany the birthing mother into the delivery suite while the men remain outside, just popping in for updates. But they never stay long. It's in and out, in and out, all day. Whoever is on reception during a Traveller birth gets a good arm workout because they are forever buzzing the men in and out. Meanwhile, it gets very crowded and noisy in the delivery suite, what with all the grandmothers, aunties, sisters and daughters chatting, fighting and giving their opinion. It's like a giant family outing. Normally our unit allows only two birthing partners, but we have to make an exception for the Travelling community, because they just won't do things any other way. Occasionally, it does mean raising my voice: 'Right, stop now. Stop talking, please! Everyone be quiet because she really needs to listen to me!'

One time we had a Traveller lady who went into labour earlier than expected. Even though she was registered at another hospital, she was in our area when her waters broke, so she rocked up at our unit, accompanied by the whole shebang. Eight caravans were parked on the grass verge outside our hospital! It was quite a sight, and they were there for three days, causing a bit of an uproar with the management. But they were a lovely, lovely family. And, as always, the men were so respectful. Traveller men treat us so well it's like something from a former era. They call us 'Nurse' or 'Sister', and every time they pop by, they shower us with flowers and chocolates.

'Here you go, Nurse. A little something for you. For doing such a grand job there.'

'Oh, that's very kind. Thank you.'

'No, thank *you*, Sister!'

'You can call me Pippa.'

'You're alright, Nurse.'

I did a few stints in the community in my early years and I had one area that included a static caravan site for Travelling families. There were about twelve caravans on this one enclosed site and despite everything I thought I knew – or the prejudices some people have – about Travellers, it was a real eye-opener to visit them in their homes. Every single one was absolutely pristine. It was immaculate, like walking into a show home. Even the children looked perfect! And they were so nicely spoken and well mannered. It definitely changed my opinion about the Travelling community and the way I approached people in general.

* * *

After a few years, I settled down in the labour ward at the hospital. Generally, I preferred the excitement of delivering babies every day to working in the community. And though I enjoyed looking after pregnant women and visiting new mums, the lure of the hospital always drew me back. I was constantly learning on the job, and not just medically. I quickly discovered that different cultures demand different considerations.

It is vital that all our mothers feel as at ease as possible during the birthing process, so, for example, when I'm dealing with a woman who is a strict Muslim, I'll be careful to make sure she is fully covered throughout. They often give birth in a full burqa, only lifting the hem when it's time to push.

For some strictly observant Muslim families, bathing the baby as early as possible is important in order to conduct prayers, whispering words in the baby's ear soon after it's born. The advice from NICE is to not bath a baby for the first five days, as the vernix – the white oily coating on their skin, which they are born with – is a natural moisturiser and should be absorbed into the skin. They argue that by washing the vernix away, we could be exposing the child to irritants or conditions like eczema. But to Muslim families, bathing the baby is part of their religious ritual. One mother had had an emergency C-section for her first child and the baby went to the neonatal unit for the first three weeks. There was no washing, which meant they couldn't do the prayers until the baby was three weeks old. For her second child, she was coming in for an induction, and the father was by her side when they asked me if they would be allowed to wash their child straight away.

'Of course you can,' I replied. 'It's your baby. This is our advice, but if you want to bathe him, that's fine. I'm not going to stop you from washing your baby.' They were so grateful, and I felt on this occasion it was important to give them back that sense of control. We have our NICE advice but, at the same time, we have to accommodate different wishes.

The one area that is very tricky is FGM – female genital mutilation. I have only come across a handful of cases of

FGM in my career. These cases are always difficult because the women are left with only a small vaginal opening, so quite often they will tear very badly. Even an intimate piercing is classed as FGM, but that doesn't need to be reported to the police. All other cases of FGM, or female circumcision, as it was previously termed, are illegal in this country. It is classed as child abuse, because it is mostly conducted on girls before they are fifteen years old – in other words, before puberty. We don't tend to find out about it until a woman is due to give birth. Then the pregnant woman will most likely confide in the community midwife, but the physical experience is not always the same. In some cases the female genital parts are still present; they have just been stitched together. But at the more extreme end of the mutilation, everything has been taken away: her labia, clitoris, everything. All that's left is a smooth area and a very small opening for the vagina. I feel terribly sorry for these women because I know it was forced upon them when they were just children. They had no choice in the matter, and the consequence is they will derive no pleasure at all from sex. Which, I suppose, is the whole point. It seems peculiarly cruel.

In FGM cases, doctors prefer to take the lead because it's harder for the birthing mother to push out the baby, and they will often need medical intervention. If the doctors are male, however, that can be problematic with the husbands. We do try and facilitate requests but there is only so much that can be done if there are no female doctors attending on the day. Occasionally, we have to be quite stern and tell the father that either he lets a doctor do his job or he needs to leave. It is quite maddening at times to see how people will put religious belief above medical necessity. Sometimes

I just want to scream at them: 'If you don't let this doctor help, the next time you see him, it will be to pronounce your baby dead!' But I'm pretty sure such vocal persuasion wouldn't fall within NHS or NICE guidelines.

If an FGM victim tears during labour, which is highly likely, then our doctors are forbidden from sewing her back up the way she came into the unit. She has to be repaired as a normal vagina would be repaired and allowed to heal normally. Even if we know she is then likely to go elsewhere and be sewn back up the way she was. It's heartbreaking, and I'll never understand how anybody can believe that a god wishes these women to be disfigured and scarred in such a way. But we don't make any comment or judgement in the room. Whatever happens, we stay respectful and professional throughout. Of course, there are plenty of times when we also deal with women who can't speak to us, as there is a language barrier. In these circumstances, we can get a translator in, but the truth is language isn't always necessary. I've found, in my line of work, we are all capable of communicating with one another as human beings. You don't need words to express pain, fear, joy or despair. You can see it in a woman's eyes. I can tell a woman to 'push' and she knows what I'm saying, even if she doesn't have the words.

Whatever the situation I find myself in, I always do my best for every woman that comes onto the ward because, in the end, even though there are differences between us, I believe there is more that unites than divides us. We're all human beings; we all feel the same emotions and deserve the same respect. So, yes, I might be a chameleon on the surface, but underneath beats the same compassionate heart.

7

Catch!

'It was a roller disco,' explained Jane, the receptionist on the desk, as she scrolled through the pictures on her phone from her hen night the previous Saturday. Sadly, I'd missed it, as I was working, but since we were having a calm moment on the ward it was a chance to have a quick catch-up. *Calm* – that's the word we use. We never say 'quiet' because that's a jinx.

'So, after a few shots,' Jane went on, 'I couldn't stay on my bloody feet! I spent more time on my arse than actually roller-skating.'

She stopped scrolling at a picture of herself spread-eagled on the floor, legs in the air, her bride's veil askew, clearly the worse for wear and laughing her head off.

'That's brilliant!' I giggled. 'I bet you've got a few bruises now, though.'

'A few? I considered taking myself to A&E the morning after! I've got one on my left thigh that I swear is the size of a–'

Just then, the double doors banged open and a rather panicked-looking medical student charged in.

'Delivery . . . ah . . . er . . . I think someone's delivering out there. She might need some help,' he spluttered.

'Out where?' I asked.

'Erm . . . the corridor. She's having a baby in the corridor.'

I knew it was too bloody calm. I pressed the emergency buzzer, shouted, 'Corridor delivery!' and jumped into action.

I ran into the corridor just in time to see a man trying to pull his wife out of the lift where she remained, on all fours, clearly in the later stages of labour. Several more midwives followed me out. All of us could see straight away there was no way we could move her.

'Right, someone's delivering here,' I announced to the assembled onlookers in the corridor. 'Can we clear some space, give this lady a little privacy, please.' One of my colleagues stood at the lift and barred anyone from getting in or out, while another secured the staircase. The rest of the team formed a protective human barrier around the woman to give her a little dignity. I bent down next to her.

'What's your name, love?'

'Liz,' she puffed.

'Okay, Liz. We're all here, we're all midwives, and no one else can see in. It looks like you're having your baby right now, so we're going to have to get your trousers off. Alright?'

She nodded wordlessly as her face contorted with pain and she bore down hard. I ripped down her trousers and knickers and thank God I did! The baby's head was already half out and the rest of the body slid out almost immediately into my arms.

Catch!

'He's here, Liz!' I gasped. 'Your baby's arrived. He's a boy, a lovely little boy.'

Just then the man next to me whispered, 'He's my son! My son!' Then he started to laugh and cry at the same time. 'I can't believe it. I can't . . . thank you. Thank you.'

I put the baby straight onto the mother's chest while the team organised a trolley to get her out of the corridor and into the delivery suite, and after all the drama was over none of us could stop smiling. That's what it's like on a labour ward – calm one minute, crazy the next.

Some babies just deliver themselves, and no matter how much planning or preparation you put in they turn up in the most unexpected places – in car parks, at home, in shopping centres or toilets. Toilets are a surprisingly common place in which to give birth because squatting is a good position for pushing. Most of the time we catch them – only once have I had to actually fish a baby out of the toilet. The woman had had an induction and the labour progressed very quickly. The baby literally just plopped into the bowl and I scooped her out, gave her a good rub down – with the famous old-fashioned NHS towel rub – and placed her straight onto Mum. No harm done!

During one birth, I asked a lady to sit on the toilet to give me a wee sample when she was in the advanced stages of labour, placing a cardboard sample pot underneath her to catch the urine.

'I'm trying but I can't wee,' she said after a little while, not even realising she was pushing. *Hmmm . . . it's working and she's coping well with the pain,* I thought. *I'll leave her on here a bit longer.*

'That's alright,' I said. 'You just stay there a few minutes and we'll see how it goes.'

I returned five minutes later and she shook her head. 'No, nothing. I'm trying but I still can't wee.' She was happy sitting there, with her partner sat in front of her, holding her hand.

'Alright, well, let's give it another five minutes,' I said, and left her alone again. She was there a good fifteen minutes, and each time I came in I could see the urge to push growing stronger and stronger. This last time, I said, 'I'll stay with you. Are you alright here?'

I didn't need to say anything or encourage her one bit. She was pushing without even realising.

'I'll tell you what, if you can stand up a little bit I'll take a look with my torch,' I suggested.

Now she stood.

'I can see your baby!' I sang out.

'What? NO!'

'Yes! It's coming.'

'In here? Now?'

'Yeah, just stay in here. It's fine.'

It was her first baby, but her body knew what it was doing. She had gone from 4 cms – what we call active labour – to the transition phase until she was ready to push, all within a few short hours. She stayed on that toilet and, at the moment of delivery, I put my hand underneath to catch the baby and she delivered into my arms. Neither of the parents could believe it had been so easy, and the mum didn't even realise she was delivering until the moment the baby arrived.

'I can't believe I gave birth on the toilet!' she said to me afterwards.

Catch!

'It's not that unusual,' I said smiling. Actually, it's much more common than most people realise. After all, a toilet makes sense. Gravity is on your side, it's at the right height to bear down with your feet on the floor, and there's a hole in the middle so you're not constricted down below. Quite frequently, I've had women go to the loo only to find they can't get off again.

'It's coming! It's coming!' they shout from the bathroom, and I'll have to quickly dive in and shove a towel or a pillow down the bowl. It's no coincidence that old-fashioned birthing stools looked exactly like toilets. We used to have one on the ward, but it was condemned after it got a crack in it. It didn't matter – the toilet worked best anyway.

Not long after the corridor baby incident, I attended to a woman expecting twins, who had been induced. She moved pretty quickly through the different phases until she was 10 cms, fully dilated, and we decided to move her to the delivery suite. She was coping very well with the pain on gas and air, going very quiet whenever a contraction came on, so I showed her to the delivery room before dashing off for a quick wee. It had been hours since I'd last emptied my bladder, so I was desperate. Then, while I was sat on the toilet, the emergency buzzer went. *That can't be my lady!* I thought. *Maybe it is . . .* I jumped up off the toilet mid-wee, ran outside and, sure enough, the emergency buzzer was flashing over the door of my twin lady. I ran straight in to find one of the babies' heads was out, already in her knickers. Luckily, one of the other midwives was in before me and she ripped off the lady's pants and out came these two beautiful babies. Just like that.

I was breathless with shock. *How did that happen?*

Normally, we would have everything prepared, the tray, drips, towels and instruments all laid out and ready before a woman gives birth. But there was no time for that. Some babies just turn up regardless of where you are at that moment in time, or if a midwife is anywhere nearby.

Whether birth happens on the toilet, in the car park or on the bed, it's the same normal process, just in an abnormal place. And to me, the best part is having a little squeeze with the baby afterwards. I don't care what some people say, I think all babies are beautiful. It's the newness of them that makes them so perfect, and it's not that often we get to hold them. Most people think that's all us midwives do all day – drink tea, eat cake and cuddle babies – but we don't get many cuddles. Not nearly enough as I'd like. Most of the time my job is running around like a headless chicken, fetching stuff. I'm forever running in and out of rooms, fetching drugs, doctors or drip stands. At the very end of it all, I think the least we deserve is a squeeze with a new baby!

* * *

By the age of twenty-two, I was happy and confident in my job, loving every minute I spent on the ward. I felt I was on the right path – every day I learned new techniques and skills, improving my abilities and adding to the experiences that made me a better midwife. Yes, in my working life, I had found contentment. I only wish I could have said the same for my romantic life. Rob and I had got together when we were both sixteen and still at school. Although we were really close, I wouldn't exactly call it a passionate love affair. Rob had always supported my dream of becoming a midwife, but after seven years I'd changed. I wasn't the same timid young girl he'd met when we were teenagers. And I didn't see him in the same way either. Rob worked in the IT department of a large insurance company, but he didn't have any burning love for his job. He was happy enough to clock in and clock out again. Now our relationship had settled into a regular pattern. Each night, Rob came round to my house, where my mum would cook tea, and then he'd hang around, sitting on the sofa watching TV till about 9 p.m., before kissing me on the cheek and returning home.

I'd wave him off at the door and then go out to the pub to meet my friends. It was the same every night. We were in a rut, though I would never have admitted that to myself, let alone anyone else. No, to the outside world we were as happy as we'd always been. And the reason I couldn't face the truth was that Rob and I were engaged. He had proposed a year earlier and, like a fool, I had said yes. To this day I don't know why. I probably thought it was the done thing, and I thought I loved him at the time. I certainly didn't want to hurt his feelings, and it never occurred to me to say no. This is what you did. My parents had got together when they were very young and stayed married all this time. I just assumed I was on a similar path.

Hanging out in the Queen's Head with my friends one night, I bumped into an old friend, Will. Will and I knew each other through mutual friends, and whenever we met at the pub we always had a good laugh together. He was funny and smart and, like me, he was also in a long-term relationship. I had just come from Mum's sofa, and another uninspiring evening with Rob, and I was joking around, entertaining Will with the details of my thrilling home life.

'Honestly, we're like Denise and Dave from *The Royle Family*!' I laughed. 'We just lounge on the sofa. One day, we'll get a sofa of our own and I'll have to start making him Dairy Lea dunkers, unless we just keep going round my mum's for tea. She *does* have the forty-inch screen!'

'Seriously?' Will looked sceptical. 'You don't seem like the Denise Royle sort to me. She's a right lazy cow. You're not like that at all. It sounds like you and Rob aren't right together.'

'Maybe . . .' I sighed into my vodka, lime & soda.

'Then finish it.'

'What?'

'Just finish it with him.'

'It's not that simple.'

'Yeah, it is. If he's not right for you, then you need to put yourself first. What's the point of being with him if he bores you to tears?'

'But we're engaged.'

'So? Are you really going to marry this man? What's the point? If you don't love him, just finish it. After all, if you do end up marrying him and resenting him for the rest of your life, you'll only make him miserable, too.'

'Yeah, God, that's true! I never really thought about it like that.'

I went home that night and tried to imagine my future. I thought about all the places I wanted to visit, my ambitions at work, as well as my hopes for a family of my own one day. And then I knew – my future didn't have Rob in it. He was nice enough, but he had no drive, no get up and go. I loved going out, meeting people, trying new things, but Rob was very content with a quiet life and I wasn't happy to spend the rest of my life compromising. Will had given me the kick up the bum I needed. When I finally got up the courage to break off the engagement, Rob was shocked and upset, but the person who took it worse was my mother. She was devastated.

'Are you sure?' she kept asking over and over. 'I thought you were so happy together.'

'Oh, Mum! I'm just good at putting on a face. I've not been happy with Rob for ages.'

'But we had so many nice holidays together . . .'

It was true. We had gone away with my family many times. But perhaps this was part of the problem – everything felt so comfortable; he was more like a brother to me than a lover.

'Look, just let it go, Mum. I'm not going to marry him. Bloody hell! Whose side are you on anyway?'

'Yours. Yours, of course. But, well, I just feel sorry for him.'

I had never felt better. It was like a huge weight had been lifted from my shoulders. I hadn't even realised it, but I had begun to dread Rob's nightly visits. I knew it was the right thing to do and, like Will said, when it came down to it, it was pretty simple. After all, we didn't live together and hadn't got any further in our wedding plans – we were having one of those ridiculously long engagements where we planned to get married years in advance of actually doing it. Thinking about it, I wondered if I'd been putting it off because I knew in my heart I didn't want to marry him. I was still young. He was still at home with his folks and so was I.

Now free of the routine, I went out every night, seeing different friends and enjoying my new, single life. For the next few months I let my hair down, going out on the tiles with my mates, flirting and making the most of my newfound freedom. Six months later, I was back in the Queen's Head when I bumped into Will. He said he hadn't been around much because he'd been on the road, travelling in his job as a film gaffer. We got chatting and he filled me in on all the European cities he'd visited. It was thrilling, hearing about all these different places. Meanwhile, I told him how I'd taken his advice and broken it off with Rob.

'Ah yes, the dazzling Robert. Well? Was that a good move?'

'Oh my God, *sooooo good*!'

'How did he take it?'

'He was fine, but my mother will never forgive me!' He laughed and I grinned back. For the first time, I saw that Will was quite attractive. It's funny, I'd never really thought of him in that way before. I mean, yes, I liked him, but I hadn't fancied him – until now.

'Well, aren't you going to buy me a drink?' I suggested flirtatiously.

'Aren't you going to buy me one?' he countered.

The cheek of it!

'I'll tell you what,' he said. 'We'll go in rounds.'

Rounds? What is that all about? At least he had the decency to get the first round in, and after that we chatted all night, taking it in turns to go the bar.

'Well, now you're a free woman, do you want to meet up again and go on a date?' he asked at the end of the night.

'You're with someone, aren't you?' I said.

'I'm not. We split up. She wasn't right for me.'

Catch!

And that was how it started.

Will was completely different to anyone I'd dated before. He was outgoing and adventurous, the complete opposite of my ex, and he always had something going on. A scheme, an idea, a project – he restored old furniture and classic motorbikes, and loved design and art. Being with Will was exciting. He drove me in his little vintage soft-top car to old country pubs in the middle of nowhere, where the ale was served in jugs next to a real open fire. There were homemade pork pies, scruffy dogs, men with flat caps, and cheeseboards the size of dinner trays. He'd ring me up, tell me to pack an overnight bag and whisk me away to posh hotels for amazing meals and nights away. Will was an old-fashioned gent. He liked real ale, beer festivals, fine wine, old whiskeys and good company. That might sound boring, but it wasn't, and when he took me out he treated me like a princess. We just had the best time ever. In my whole life I'd never laughed so much with somebody. We shared a love of travel, an interest in the world around us, and the same wicked sense of humour. I never realised being with someone could be so much fun. And the best thing was, I felt completely myself when I was with him. The only person who didn't seem so happy about my new romance was Mum.

'It's a bit soon, isn't it?' she scowled, when I told her I was seeing Will.

'What do you mean? It's been six months since I split up with Rob.'

'Yes, but you need time to get over it.'

'No I don't. I was the one who ended things.'

'Oh well, you know best,' she snapped sarcastically. It was

upsetting. Will hadn't done anything wrong, nor had I, and yet she was pouring a big bucket of cold water all over my happiness. It was like she felt I didn't deserve to be happy after breaking off the engagement and hurting Rob. She was even more disapproving when I announced we were taking a mini-break together, just one month after starting to date.

'I can't believe you've booked a holiday with someone you've only just met,' she said. 'Don't you think you ought to wait till you know him better?'

'Why? I know him really well already. We haven't just met. We've been friends for years.'

'Well, think about Rob, then. Don't you think it might be humiliating for him to learn you've hooked up with someone else already and now you're off gallivanting to Venice.'

'Vienna.'

'Whatever.'

'I don't see why he should have anything to say at all, Mum. I mean, what makes you think he'll even find out. Hmmm?'

It was irritating to have to keep justifying myself to her, but I suppose she'd got used to the idea of me being with Rob. Perhaps she felt guilty that he had lost *us*, his second family, and sad too that our little group for the past five years was now gone. And since I was out of the house more, too, maybe she felt she'd lost me as well. But I couldn't allow myself to worry about her feelings all the time – I was head over heels in love!

Nine months into our blossoming romance, I found out I was pregnant. It was a complete shock. I had been on the pill the whole time, but I had missed a couple of days when we went away for one or two nights. At the time, I honestly didn't think it would make a difference, but I should have known better. Now I stared in disbelief at the white stick showing two unmistakable blue lines. Of course, I had always wanted children, but now? Will and I had been together for less than a year.

Was it too soon? What would he think? What would he say? My mind raced with questions as I resolved to talk to him the next day. The only thing I knew for certain was that Mum wouldn't be happy.

8

Not Without My Baby

The next morning at work we were all called into a meeting with Social Services. This was fairly unusual. It was quite common for women who came through the ward to be involved with Social Services in some way, but we were rarely briefed in person. Usually, we read the Social Service alerts on a woman's maternity notes, but nothing so grand as a meeting.

'Okay, settle down, ladies,' urged Jen, the LWC. 'I need your full attention, please.' She waited for silence before carrying on.

'We've got a lady coming in today for an induction, as she's several days past her due date. Social Services would like to brief you about her as there's a very particular set of circumstances surrounding her case, and every single midwife on the ward needs to be aware of the situation. I'll let Carol explain the rest.'

She sat down and Carol, the Child Protection Officer from Social Services, stood up and addressed us all. She

101

explained that the woman, Charlie, would be coming in, and her unborn child was currently the subject of a protection order with a view to placing that child into immediate protective care.

'Let me just give you a little background to this case,' Carol said. 'Charlie's husband was convicted last year of multiple offences of child abuse and making pornographic images and videos of children over a number of years. He'd turned a room of his house into a photographic studio and was one of several members of a child pornography ring that operated, not just in this area, but nationwide. The police were able to identify and arrest several members of that ring, all of whom are now behind bars, having been convicted of child sexual abuse offences.

'Charlie claimed all the way through the court case that she had no idea of the crimes her husband committed in their home. She says she didn't know that the studio was used to take pictures of children. He too maintained she was innocent. Although the police weren't convinced, they could not find any evidence of her involvement. Hence, she was never charged with any offences. Before her husband was convicted, they split up. Charlie left him and that was that. End of story. And that might have been the end of our involvement with her, but last year she became romantically involved with her husband's best friend, Archie.

'Now, the police have been aware of this friend Archie since day one, and though several questions were raised about him during the course of the investigation, the CPS felt there wasn't enough evidence to bring any charges against him. And now . . . well, Charlie is pregnant with this gentleman's baby and we have great concerns about the safeguarding of this new child. Given the serious nature of the offences surrounding them, we have applied to the court for a Full Care Order and, in the interim, as soon as Charlie has given birth, an Emergency Protection Order. Charlie and Archie, however, are currently fighting the orders. The case will be heard in front of a judge as soon as the baby is born and our ducks are in a row. We've talked this over with senior management here and I think it would be best if Charlie is placed as close to the nurses' station as possible, to monitor her carefully. Any observations made may be relevant to the order, so it's vital she's watched twenty-four seven. Okay – any questions?'

I put my hand up.

'So, she's not been convicted of any crime and nor has the father?'

'That's right, but we have conducted a full risk assessment on the safeguarding of this child and we believe there are substantial reasons for concern, enough to warrant taking the child into our full protective custody.'

'So, you think this guy Archie had something to do with the child pornography ring? Or she did? Or they both did, and you just can't prove it? Is that right?'

'I didn't say that,' she returned tartly and moved onto another question.

No, but that was clearly what you implied.

After the meeting broke up, we were all curious to find out more. It was a strange situation, and though we were used to seeing babies taken from their mothers by Social Services every month or so, this was not a run-of-the-mill case by any stretch. And it certainly wasn't the norm for mothers to fight the order through the courts. If a woman was already involved with Social Services, she would usually have a good idea by the time of the birth whether she was going to be able to take her baby home. There could be a host of reasons for this, including abuse and neglect, though by far the most common reason was drug or alcohol abuse. They'd be tested throughout the pregnancy and, if the tests proved they weren't clean, the baby would be taken into foster care straight from hospital. In these events, Social Services did try to place the child with another member of the family as much as possible, although it didn't always work out that way.

Every case was different. I'd seen some babies removed for what seemed like quite minor offences from women who had clearly tried very hard to stay clean, while others were allowed to take their baby home under supervision when they had a whole list of infractions on their notes. I suppose we didn't always know the full ins and outs of the matter, only the final stages, but each time I hated it. It was horrible to have to watch the mother leave the ward without her child. We always gave them lots of time alone with their babies in those final, difficult hours. I didn't like to watch; these were very precious, private moments they were sharing, and not for the prying eyes of strangers.

Unlike what you might see on TV, there were very rarely any dramas – no big outbursts, shouting or mothers being dragged away by burly security guards. No, these were sad, solemn occasions. Most mums accepted the decision and left quietly without a word. By that point, there was a level of acceptance and understanding – they had been tested throughout the pregnancy and, if it was proven that they had fallen short, this was the outcome they had been warned of. This is what they knew to expect, so now there was no point fighting. The mother would leave the baby in our care and we would take charge of them until Social Services brought the foster carer to the ward. It was heartbreaking whenever a little baby was left alone on the ward. I just wanted to bundle them up and take them home with me.

Charlie came in just before midday. She seemed normal in every way. She was in her late twenties with dark-brown hair scraped back into a high ponytail, and she wore baggy jogging pants and a large T-shirt with the slogan 'Baby on Board'. There was nothing unusual about the way she looked: she wasn't particularly rough; she didn't have any tattoos or piercings; she wasn't odd or distinctive in any way. She was just like you and me – ordinary. Her partner, Archie, was with her for the induction and the pair seemed like any other expectant parents-to-be: happy, nervous and excited all at once. Only in this case there was another level of anticipation at the outcome of the birth: would they be allowed to keep their child?

Their solicitor joined them in the late afternoon and went through the case with them. He explained that as soon as the child was born, they would be issued with an Emergency Protection Order and given a court date to fight the Full Care Order. I felt sorry for Charlie. She seemed like a nice lady and this was her first child. If she hadn't done anything wrong, and neither had her partner, it seemed like a terrible punishment to inflict on them both. Charlie went into labour just as my shift ended.

I left the hospital and went straight round to see Will at his grandmother's house, where he was living at the time.

I was a bundle of nerves, worrying about how he would react to the news that I was pregnant. I couldn't hold back, I just came straight out with it, and was relieved when he immediately broke into a massive grin.

'Are you kidding?' he asked, smiling from ear to ear.

'No,' I laughed. 'It's true. Are you happy?'

'Yeah! Of course I am!' he said. 'I've always wanted kids, you know that.'

'I know, but is it too soon?'

'I don't think so. I think we should go for it. What do you think?'

I was flooded with relief. I knew that we were right for one another and it was so good to hear that Will felt the same.

'Yeah, I think so too. Let's go for it.'

* * *

The next day, I was in at 6.45 a.m., ready to go into handover at 7 a.m. in the side room on the ward. As usual, there were two healthcare assistants, six midwives and a couple of student midwives. The night-time coordinator came in and ran through the list of women we had on the ward, detailing who had given birth and who was in labour. Charlie had had her little girl overnight, a spontaneous vaginal birth, and both mum and baby were doing well. She gave us the details of everyone else on the ward, and we were allocated different women to look after, as well as discussing who else we were expecting to come in later in the day. I was given Charlie. The doctors were due to do their handover an hour after us, so I used that time to visit my ladies and to speak to the midwife on the previous shift for a more detailed picture of the care plan.

Charlie was bottle-feeding her little girl when I went to see her on the ward.

'Oh, she's gorgeous!' I smiled. 'How are you feeling?'

'Tired,' said Charlie. 'Tired and happy. And scared I'm going to lose her.'

I sat down on the chair next to her. My job wasn't just about looking after her physical needs; it was important to build a relationship, to gain her trust. And for that I had to know her side of things.

'Tell me about it,' I said. 'I mean, I've seen the notes from Social Services, but I want to hear your side of things. Tell me what's happening and where we're at.'

'They don't think I'm able to look after her because of what happened with my ex.' She sighed. 'The police, they tried to say that I was involved in it, but there was no proof because I'm innocent. I had no idea what was going on. I mean, it's terrible what he did to those children – it makes me feel sick – but I had nothing to do with it. Yet *I'm* the one being punished. It's not fair.'

She seemed angry, and I could see that if she was telling the truth then the actions of Social Services might seem very cruel. Officially, she hadn't done anything wrong, and yet she was being judged for what her ex-husband had done. It was guilt by association.

Charlie stayed on our ward for several days, fighting the care order through the courts. Every day, we did a full check-up on her and her baby and she'd wander round the ward, getting bottles from the station and bringing us up to date on the progress of her case. I had a lot of sympathy for her situation. Social Services said that if Archie wasn't involved then things might be different, but they didn't give any guarantees of dropping the order if she left him. They argued that her choice of men proved that she lacked judgement and could not be trusted to protect her child. Charlie, however, was adamant that they were both innocent and were being treated unfairly just because of her ex-husband's actions. As the father of the baby, she said Archie had every right to be involved with the care of their child. Every day she had to attend court, and though it was a wrench for her to leave her baby on the ward, I could see the determination in her eyes – it was the determination of a mother who would do anything for their child. *Was she really capable of putting this child in harm's way?* I wondered. On the other hand, all those other children had been harmed right under her nose, so was she capable of protecting any child?

From what I observed on the ward, Charlie was a natural mother, caring for her baby beautifully, attending to her when she cried, feeding her, putting her down to sleep and changing her when she needed a new nappy. And she seemed so happy around her child. It brought up so many questions in my mind. *Didn't Charlie have the right to move on with her life and start a new family? Was there more to it that I wasn't aware of?* It went against all my natural instincts to force this woman apart from her child, especially when they were clearly so bonded. On the other hand, observing a woman on the ward wasn't the same as seeing her in her everyday life. Who knew what could happen if she was allowed to take the baby home? But what effect would it have on Charlie if she was denied the chance of having her own family? It all made my head spin! This was a huge, life-changing decision for everyone involved and I didn't envy the judge one bit.

On the final court date, Charlie came back to the ward in

a state of emotional distress. It was clear she had lost her appeal. That was a terrible day – she kept breaking down in tears the whole time, not wanting to leave, telling us how difficult it was, the thought of leaving her little girl in hospital and never coming back.

'What's she going to think of me when she grows up and hears all about her real mum? She'll think I've abandoned her!' she wept.

'No, no,' I soothed. 'She wouldn't think that, not after everything you've done to try and keep her.'

'But how will she know? Who's going to tell her?'

We gave her all the time and privacy she needed to make those final few hours together as special as possible, but time was no friend to Charlie, and it wasn't long before she had to leave. Her eyes were so full of sadness I could barely look at them.

'I'll never give up,' she said, shaking with emotion. 'I'll never give up fighting for her. Never.'

'I know, Charlie, I know,' I said, fighting back my own tears.

'I'll get her back. I will. I'll get her back.'

Charlie stopped then and looked at me: 'Thank you, Pippa. Thank you for not judging me.'

We hugged and I whispered, 'Look after yourself.'

She nodded, and then quietly she took Archie's hand and together they slipped away. In the corner of the room her baby girl softly slept. And maybe it was the fine balance of the decision about Charlie's baby, the courage she showed in fighting for her child, or my own pregnancy, but I ached for Charlie's loss.

* * *

We try not to judge the women and girls that come through our doors. That's not our job. Our job is to make their transition to motherhood as smooth as possible, and to give them the tools and confidence to go away and care for their newborn baby. It's not always straightforward. Sometimes, they come to us not even realising they're about to give birth. Very often, the young ones – twelve-, thirteen-, fourteen-year-olds – they'll arrive on the ward unbooked, not even realising they're pregnant. They appear at A&E with abdominal pains, claiming not to know they are nine months pregnant.

Sometimes you believe them and sometimes you don't. For some girls, it's clear they have a bump they've been hiding under big, layered clothes, but if they're very young and their muscle tone is good, they might not have big bumps at all. We have to exercise our judgement – in most of these cases, we'll have to inform Social Services because, after all, a child having a child is evidence of a crime. Then someone from Social Services will come to the hospital and that girl won't be allowed to leave with her baby until they have a care plan in place to work out whether she is capable of looking after it. Does she have the right support in place? What about the family?

We play a crucial role in this assessment: the girls talk to us and we get as much information as possible, which we share with Social Services. It is up to us to observe how they manage in the first few hours or days with their baby. Does it look like the new mum is bonding with her baby? Is she getting as much support as she needs? Does she have a stable home to return to? Though we see many young girls on our ward, I'm continually amazed by their ability to cope with the rigors of childbirth. They just do it! It's as if they let their bodies take over and they give birth without much fuss.

Many of the families get on with it, too. One sixteen year old came in with abdominal pains and we had to inform both her and her family that she was in labour. They didn't have a clue she was pregnant and, consequently, they had nothing prepared at home. But after the girl gave birth, the mum went straight out to Mothercare and came back an hour later with everything she would need for the baby: car seat, nappies, sleepsuits, bottles, steriliser, the lot! And then they all trotted off home with this baby as if it was the most natural thing in the world – which, of course, it was.

We don't always have to inform the authorities. I live and work in a fairly deprived area, so we have a high teen-pregnancy rate. It's normal around here for a fifteen-year-old to come in and have a baby. And, as long as it's consensual, that doesn't give us any cause for concern. Of course, it's a different matter if the girls are twelve or thirteen, but we've got very used to seeing eighteen-year-olds coming into hospital on their third or fourth pregnancy. It has become a way of life for some people, one that is repeated down the generations. Quite often, the mother of the teenager has had her children young, too, and we meet plenty of grandmothers in their early thirties.

One time, we had a woman who became a grandmother at the age of twenty-six. I never met her, but everyone on the unit was discussing her case because, well, that's definitely out of the ordinary. And whatever you think about Social Services, the organisation plays a crucial role in supporting young families when they have no other means of support.

For example, if a woman comes in without a home to go back to, Social Services will put her in a mother and baby unit until they can sort her out with a home. They help people when they need help most.

However, there's no denying that, for some people, involvement with Social Services has not been a positive experience and occasionally this leads to drastic action. One lady with a long history of drug abuse had had two children taken from her. We didn't even know she was pregnant again until we got the emergency call at midnight requesting the attendance of a midwife to an allotment on the outskirts of town.

'What? Can you say that again?' I asked Ambulance Control on the phone.

'We have a lady in a tent on the allotment next to the bypass, just outside of town. She's in labour and in considerable distress. Are you able to send a midwife?'

'Yes, of course,' I replied, as Helen, one of the most senior members of our team, flung on her coat and I handed her the details of her destination.

'Good luck!' I mouthed. She gave me the thumbs-up and ran out. Later, she filled me in on the details. This mum, a former heroin addict, had concealed her pregnancy in a bid to keep her baby – no scans, no antenatal care, nothing. Her plan was to give birth in secret and keep the child away from health professionals until she moved out of the area. But the moment she went into labour, she realised she couldn't do it alone. She panicked and dialled 999, and it's a jolly good thing she did because, when Helen went to assist, she found she wasn't delivering just one baby but two!

'So, there I am, kneeling on all fours, half in, half out of this bloody tiny tent, juggling a baby in each arm, trying to keep them warm while the mother delivers the placenta,' she said. I had to admire Helen; she was such a pro.

'I mean, forget Bear Grylls, this was *Extreme Midwifing*,' she said, sighing.

'Hmm. *Giving Birth in the Wild*? I think it would be a hit show,' I mused.

'I thought of it first!'

9

Born Too Soon

'I've had a baby and it's dead,' the woman said, slowly and deliberately. I was on Reception, filling out some paperwork when the young woman walked in carrying a plastic bag, accompanied by an older and frail-looking lady. The younger woman looked to be in her mid-twenties, wore loose baggy joggers, no make-up, and her greasy, loose brown hair fell in a messy bob around her shoulders. The old lady next to her wore a blue mac and a worried expression. They both seemed normal enough, but there was something in the slow, monotone delivery of the young woman, and the way her eyes were fastened on the floor, that told me she probably had some kind of disability. And what she had said was just plain odd.

'I'm sorry, what do you mean?' I asked her.

'I've brought it in with me.' And with that she lifted up a well-worn Tesco Bag for Life and plonked it down on the desk. There was something in the shape and weight of the contents of the bag that struck an instant chill within me.

The Secret Midwife

Dear God, I hope that's not what I think it is.

'Erm, what's in the bag?' I asked cautiously, my heart now thumping in my chest.

'It's the baby,' she said simply, and the old lady next to her nodded sadly and murmured, 'The baby.'

I exchanged a look with Helen, who was sitting on the desk with me.

'I didn't know . . .' the woman started to say, looking down at the desk. 'But then I was on the toilet and it just came out. And I saw it was a baby, but it wasn't moving or crying or nothing, so my grandma said we'd better go to the hospital. So we got it out the toilet and put it in the bag and then we got on the number forty-three bus and then we had to change buses – to the number twenty-seven, I think . . . yes, the number twenty-seven. And that's how we came here. But I don't know why a baby has come out . . . I just don't know.'

'It's alright, love,' said her grandmother, now offering comfort by stroking her arm, nicotine-stained fingers contrasting with her royal-blue sweatshirt.

'You don't know why a baby has come out?' I asked, trying to grasp this unbelievable situation.

'I don't know why it's happened because I've never had sex with anyone. I'm a virgin.'

At that, Helen took in a deep breath and her eyebrows shot up. *Bloody hell!*

'Right, well, since you've had a baby, we'd better make sure you're alright,' I said. 'What's your name?'

'It's Sally. Sally Anne Hughes and I am twenty-eight,' she said very slowly. 'And I've got learning disabilities.'

She said those last two words extra slowly, careful not

to stumble, but without a hint of embarrassment or self-consciousness. She was clearly used to telling people about her challenges.

'Yes, she's got learning disabilities,' her grandmother repeated. 'And she lives with me.'

'So, I don't understand everything too well,' Sally went on.

'But she knows she's had a baby,' her grandmother interjected.

'I mean, I do understand lots of things. I work in a Sue Ryder shop,' Sally went on.

'That's right.' Her grandmother nodded again, and Sally concluded, 'But not all things. I don't understand *all* things. Am I in trouble?'

There was a pause now as both women looked at me.

'It's okay, Sally,' I said, smiling. 'You're not in trouble, sweetheart, so don't worry. Your grandmother was right to bring you here. This hospital is the best place for you and your baby, and we are going to look after you. Now, this lady called Helen here will take you down to one of our rooms to have a quick look at you and make sure everything is okay. And I'll stay here and look after your baby, shall I?'

The woman nodded and Helen led her away while I carefully picked up the bag from the counter. I found a quiet room and carefully placed it on a trolley. I eased my hands into some surgical gloves and, after pulling out my scissors, I began to cut at the old plastic bag with slow rhythmic precision, every snip bringing me closer to its grim contents. Inside was the cold, still, lifeless body of a baby boy that looked to be around twenty-four weeks. Using both hands, I scooped up his tiny floppy body, placed him onto a towel and started to take his measurements.

117

All the while my head swam. I could hardly believe he'd been carried here on two buses in a plastic carrier bag. A Bag for *bloody* Life of all things! How did those two women sit there with that bag on the floor next to them? Next to other passengers! It was just surreal. The baby was small enough to fit in my hands when both cupped; his eyes were fused shut, and his cold, red skin was translucent and shiny. Otherwise, he was normal – like a miniature version of a fully grown baby.

I called the paediatrician, who confirmed that Sally had experienced a late miscarriage. That jarred with me. I hated calling a well-developed baby a 'late miscarriage' – it felt like such a cold, clinical description. After all, if it had been a couple of weeks later, we would have termed the child *stillborn*. Actually, he might well have been over twenty-four weeks – we couldn't tell the exact age, because Sally hadn't realised she was pregnant, so she hadn't had any check-ups or midwife visits.

She said he had been born showing no signs of life, and yet there was no clear reason we could see why the child had died, although we only had her words to go on. The whole thing was a mystery. Meanwhile, Helen found the cord had snapped inside Sally, so she had to help her to deliver the placenta by giving her an injection of oxytocin into her leg and clamping the broken end of the cord and applying gentle traction. She bled a little more than we would have liked during this procedure, so we decided to keep her in for observation, and to give us time to call Social Services. From everything that she was telling us, we had plenty of reasons to be concerned.

'I just don't know how I could have a baby,' Sally repeated

when I saw her on the ward. She was still in a state of shock – not emotional in the least, just bewildered and incredulous. I pulled up a chair next to her bed and I asked her what she meant.

'I mean, I never actually had sex with him,' she said. 'I told you – I'm a virgin.'

'Sex with who?' I probed gently.

'With John, my boyfriend. I met him in the shop, in the Sue Ryder shop.'

It was a slow process but I gradually got to the bottom of Sally's bizarre story. She explained that she volunteered two days a week at her local charity shop and John had been a regular customer who seemed to pay her special attention. When he'd asked her out on a date, she had readily agreed, though she was quick to point out that at fifty-five, he was quite a bit older than her.

'It was nice,' she said. 'He took me to the café in the park, and to the community cinema and to Gala Bingo. I like bingo.'

Sally admitted that John had stayed over at her grand-mother's house a couple of times, but they had only kissed and 'done other sexy things'. Although she was absolutely adamant they had never slept together. It was all very strange. To my mind, there were only three possible explanations: one, she didn't know what sex actually meant; two, she had consented to sex and then forgotten or blanked the incident from her mind; or three, a more sinister explanation, was that she was telling the truth and John had drugged and raped her without her consent. Either way, she was a vulnerable person in a very difficult situation.

'Are you still with John?' I asked. 'Is he still your boyfriend?'

'No!' she replied fiercely. 'No way. I don't like him any more. He's a sicko.'

Now things took an even darker twist. Sally clammed up and wouldn't say any more, but her grandmother explained that the day before the miscarriage, John had been exposed by a group of vigilante paedophile hunters. The group had created a fake profile for a twelve-year-old girl whom John had communicated with in an online chatroom. They had arranged to meet up, but when John went to meet 'her' in the local park, the group confronted him on camera, streaming this live on social media. The film had been passed to the police, who later arrested John and charged him with Solicitation of a Minor. It was the police who had called Sally and informed her of John's arrest. According to her grandmother, she then 'lost it', crying and shouting and getting very upset. Hours later, she started to bleed. It led me to wonder whether the physical shock of the exposé had brought on the miscarriage. We relayed all this to Social Services, who came to see Sally and her grandmother in hospital, and the police arrived to take a statement later that day.

I had dressed Sally's baby and placed him in a cool cot in the corner of her room. At first, she didn't seem very interested in the child. It was almost like he wasn't there. But every now and again her eyes were drawn to the cot in the corner, curiosity got the better of her, and she would ask me if she could have a look at him.

'Of course you can,' I'd say. 'He's your baby.'

She'd nod solemnly, get up off the bed and wander over to the cot, then stand there for several minutes, just looking down, frowning at her baby and biting her nails. It was like she couldn't quite believe he was hers. Then she'd go back and sit on her bed without a word. An hour later, she'd ask me again: 'Can I look at him?'

The next day, the bereavement midwife went to speak to Sally and her grandmother about counselling. Sally said that she understood but she wasn't interested in having counselling, thanks, and, quite frankly, since she didn't know she was having a baby, she didn't feel sad that the baby was dead. I suppose that even after a day or two the whole thing seemed too far-fetched for her to take on board. According to her she had literally experienced a virgin birth. Together, Sally and her grandmother settled on a hospital-arranged cremation, which was the simplest funeral to organise. It was also free and the only thing you had to pay for were the flowers, if you wanted any, which Sally didn't. Neither did she want to name her baby, so the hospital issued a cardboard coffin emblazed with one simple word: 'Infant'. Two days later, Sally and her grandmother left hospital with Sally determined never to date an older man again.

* * *

Though Sally's case had been one of the strangest I'd ever been involved with, miscarriages are all too common in my line of work. The fact is that one in four pregnancies ends in miscarriage, so this is something you get used to dealing with. And sadly some occur very late in pregnancy, but up until twenty-four weeks there's nothing we can do. The advice and policies from the NHS, NICE, the Royal College of Obstetricians and Gynaecologists (RCOG) and the British Medical Association (BMA) currently state that if a baby is born before that time it is just too small to attempt resuscitation – although this is under review at the time of writing. They are not considered 'viable'. It's not the same in all countries – you hear stories from abroad of babies born as young as twenty-one or twenty-two weeks surviving, but we have our guidelines and there's simply no room for manoeuvre. It's heartbreaking, but I have been in the room when a baby is born just under twenty-four weeks and the family beg the paediatrician to do something, but they will not attempt resuscitation at this age, and will have to say, very firmly: 'I'm really sorry, there's nothing we can do.'

Can you imagine how hard that must be for the family? I can see the desperation in their eyes, and I understand, I truly do. I would be the same. But in the end, they always respect the paediatricians. Despite their pain, they trust the judgement of the medical professionals. But it can be a very close call. That line between life and death is so thin sometimes, it almost melts away – and then there is real confusion over what it means to be a 'viable baby'.

I had just come on shift one day when I was given a lady whose waters had gone at twenty weeks. If the waters break at twenty weeks, there is no way that baby will survive to term, so this is technically classed as a *late miscarriage.*

Eleanor had been in since lunchtime with a few pains and cramps, but by the time I walked into the room at 7.45 p.m., she was already fully dilated. Within half an hour, she delivered what she was expecting to be a stillborn baby. However, to my amazement, the baby was born alive. He was moving and had a heartbeat.

'Your baby's moving,' I said to Eleanor in astonishment. 'He's alive. Do you want to hold him?'

'No, I can't.' She seemed frightened.

'But he's your baby.'

'No . . . no!'

She wouldn't even look at him, let alone hold him. What could I do? I wrapped this baby carefully in a towel, pressed the buzzer for assistance, and, when my colleague Sam came in, I asked her to take over with the mum. Then I sat in a quiet room and held this little boy in my arms until he slowly slipped away, his tiny little body too precious for this world.

At that gestation, we couldn't have offered any resuscitation – our machines just aren't designed for babies that small – but the will to live is strong. And this child had fought so hard to get this far – to survive, to breathe, just to keep going – I couldn't bring myself to put him down to die on his own. I felt the least he deserved was to know the warmth and comfort of another human being. I wasn't his mother, but in his first and last minutes on this earth, I needed to show him love, so I held him. And gradually his breathing became fainter and shallower until it gently and quietly stopped. I looked at this perfect still baby nestled into me, as if seeking comfort from my soul to his, and without warning tears began to cascade down my face. I just sat there convulsing with muffled sobs, kissed my finger, placed it on his forehead, and cried my heart out.

Something had happened just a few days earlier. I'd been experiencing cramps and some light bleeding in the morning, so I'd gone into hospital for a scan.

'It looks fine, everything's normal,' the doctors reassured me. 'It looks to me like you're around five or six weeks. Is that right?'

'No, I thought it was more than that,' I replied. 'I'm about nine weeks by now.'

'No, you can't be,' the sonographer replied. 'The measurements would be much bigger. We've done your bloods and your hormone levels would definitely be higher if you were nine weeks. No, I'm pretty sure you're at the five- to six-week mark. Maybe you've got your dates muddled up.'

'Hmmm . . . maybe,' I scowled, unconvinced. *I'm sure I've got the right dates.* It's pretty obvious when you're ovulating, and even though we hadn't planned the pregnancy, I was sure I was nine weeks pregnant. That evening I went back to Will's house. We had just put a deposit down on our first house together and now our nights were spent poring over catalogues and websites, choosing beds, sofas and curtains. But as the evening wore on, the cramps in my stomach got worse and worse, and the pain spread to my back. The bleeding too got heavier and heavier. At 11 p.m., I went to the toilet, and that's when I passed a couple of clots. My heart sunk. I was having a miscarriage.

'It's come away,' I told Will sadly when I came out of the toilet. 'The baby. I think it's come away.'

He came up to me and gave me a cuddle and I wept heavily into his arms. *Why? Why have I lost the baby?* Even though I knew all the facts about pregnancy, that one in four ends in miscarriage, I couldn't help feeling cheated. *I'm a midwife, for God's sake, this is my profession. I've delivered hundreds of babies. I've helped hundreds of women give birth. Don't I deserve a baby too?*

I couldn't help it. Even though it hadn't been planned, the moment I'd found out I was pregnant, I had started to picture the baby and the life we would have together. I had never been pregnant before now, and I had got carried away with the possibilities. Now I wondered if I would ever be able to carry to full term. For the next day or so, I was angry with the world, that terrible question spinning round and round in my head: *Why me?*

It was so early in the pregnancy, we hadn't yet told anyone, so now I found I had no one to talk to about the miscarriage. The trouble was that Will didn't say much either. It was infuriating; he just carried on as if nothing had happened. I think he was afraid of upsetting me, but his silence was more hurtful than anything else. *Wasn't he upset, too? Didn't he care?* Gradually, the anger faded and the rational part of my brain took over again. I talked it over with the obstetrician and I began to see the signs had been there from the start. I was convinced my dates were right, which meant the foetus probably wasn't developing properly, and that might explain why my pregnancy hormones were low, too. I had to accept that the pregnancy simply wasn't meant to be.

Now I placed this dead baby back in its cot and left the room. At first, it had baffled me when Eleanor had refused to hold her baby, but the more I thought about it, the more I realised it had been fear holding her back. She was afraid to feel anything for the baby because she knew it wouldn't live. The fear of loving a dying child was just too much. But they're still babies, at the end of the day, every single one of them. And to me they're all perfect. Later, I went to see Eleanor and she asked to see her little boy.

I brought him in, and the moment she saw him she reached out her arms. It was a sweet and tender moment to see mother and son reunited; to see all that fear melt away, replaced by love, sadness and regret.

'He was going to be called Kieran,' she said quietly, tracing a finger over his nose and mouth.

'It's a lovely name,' I said. 'It suits him.'

'I'm sorry. I'm so sorry,' she wept, as she held him.

'He wasn't alone,' I said softly. 'I was with him the whole time.'

Once she had overcome her fear, Eleanor was ready to deal with the grief of losing her child. But I understood why she had shut down. I think that's how a lot of people react to difficult emotions – they cut themselves off.

I struggled with Will's buttoned-up reaction to our miscarriage. He seemed to act as if nothing was wrong. Meanwhile, I was mourning the loss of all those dreams and expectations I already had for our child, and the life we would have shared together. One night we went out to the pub to meet some friends and, by the time I got home, I was a mess: drunk, angry and tearful. Will tried cheering me up by cracking a few jokes but I wasn't in the mood to be cheered.

Eventually, I erupted: 'Stop it with the jokes. I'm sad, Will! I'm sad because of the miscarriage and that's *normal*. It's normal to be sad. You don't need to try and jolly me up. What's not normal is pretending like it doesn't fucking matter.'

'I'm not pretending,' he shot back.

'Oh really? So you honestly don't care, then? You honestly think that it doesn't matter? I suppose that means you never really wanted our baby.' For a moment, Will looked stunned, as if I had slapped him. My words brought tears to his eyes.

'I did! Don't say that. Don't you ever fucking say that! I *did* want our baby. I still do . . .' And he crumbled, sliding down the wall to the floor. Finally I had broken through the tough-guy act. I went over to where he sat, head in hands sobbing. I sat down next to him, placed my head on his shoulder and we cried together.

It's funny the walls we build to protect ourselves from pain. Sometimes those walls are helpful, and sometimes they only serve to lock us out of our real emotions and prevent us from engaging with life. We do it all the time in so many different ways. I'd seen it in the mother who had refused to hold her baby. Fear had stopped her from feeling. I wondered sometimes if this was true for my mum too. I knew that deep down she *wanted* to be happy for me; I knew she *wanted* to be hopeful, but for so many years she had been the person I had relied on for guidance, love and support. As she constantly reminded me, she only ever had my best interests at heart. Now I was going out in the world – falling in love, buying a house, going on mini-breaks – making all these big decisions without her, and she feared that without her guidance and support I would stumble and make the wrong choices. Her fear stopped her from sharing my happiness. But I was enjoying life – and even if I was making mistakes, they were mine to make. I would always need my mother in my life, but I was more than ready to move forward on my own terms.

10

Waters Waters Everywhere!

I don't know who felt more uncomfortable: the woman crouching on all fours on the trolley, or me, crouching behind her with my hand and forearm deep in her vagina, as we shot down the corridor together. Actually, at this point, it didn't matter how either of us felt. What was important was getting to theatre as quickly as possible without me taking my hand away. It might have looked odd to any casual bystander who spied us as we trundled down the corridor, but this really was a matter of life or death.

'MIND YOUR BACKS PLEASE!' shouted one of the four members of the team, two of whom were coasting us with speed as the other two jogged alongside. 'Watch your backs!'

It had been a fairly normal birth until about five minutes ago. Abi was on her second child and was having an induction. After she had been given the propess pessary to get her going, I ruptured her membranes to increase her contractions. And that's when I saw it – the cord! Now, a cord is not something you want to see before a woman has delivered her baby. It generally only happens with women who have the condition polyhydramnios, which is the fancy medical term for 'too much waters'. Usually, we would notice this on a woman's scans, but Abi hadn't had a scan since twenty weeks, so it wasn't picked up. If we had known about the polyhydramnios, we would have performed an artificial rupture of membrane (ARM), which is where we break the waters with the doctors present.

An excess of amniotic fluid means the baby has too much room to move around in the womb, and they end up in all sorts of odd positions. So, when the amniotic sac breaks it can lead to a 'cord prolapse', which is when the cord shoots down the birth canal and comes out first. This is bad. Very bad. You do not want to see cord under any circumstances, because if the cord has prolapsed, the baby's head will be coming down after it, squashing the cord and potentially cutting off the blood supply to the baby, starving it of oxygen. It's a very dangerous complication. That's why, if we know a woman has polyhydramnios, we'll try to keep her on the unit and induce her as soon as the head drops into the pelvis. And if at any point we see a cord during the birth, we know that woman needs an instant C-section (unless birth is imminent). Meanwhile, our main job is to hold the baby's head off the cord.

I had just ruptured Abi's membranes when the long loop of cord dropped down and my heart jumped into my mouth. Abi was lying flat on the bed, so my hand shot into her straight away to lift the head off the cord. I asked her partner to press the emergency buzzer. My hand was on the baby's head, pushing it back in to take the pressure off the cord. And that's how I had to stay until the consultant had the baby safely out.

'Are you okay?' I called out to Abi.

'Yeah, yeah . . . what's going on?'

'You've got a cord prolapse,' I explained. 'The cord presented first, so now it's important I keep my hand on the baby's head, up and off the cord to ensure it doesn't cut off the blood supply. We're going to have to go straight to theatre for a caesarean section to deliver your baby safely. Is that okay?'

'Okay, okay . . .' Abi seemed calm and controlled. 'As long as the baby's safe.'

'That's right. We'll do everything we can to keep the baby safe, Abi.'

I now climbed onto the bed, one-handed, so both of us were flipped onto all fours (well, I was on all threes) and down we rolled to theatre together like that, my hand wedged firmly into Abi's cervix. The team worked quickly and efficiently around us, covering us in surgical drapes while the anaesthetist administered a spinal. Abi was now lying on her back with a screen in front of her while I sat at the end of the bed, leaning in with my arm forward, covered in the hot, heavy drapes. As the lights were directed at me, I felt the damp patches under my arms growing larger and my forehead bead with sweat. Surrounded by the drapes and lights, I was beginning to feel claustrophobic, as if I might faint.

'Sheila!' I whispered to the healthcare assistant next to me. '*Psst* . . . Sheila!'

'Pippa? Is that you?' She couldn't see me under the drapes but she recognised my voice.

'Yeah. Look, I'm melting under here. Would you do me a favour, please? Get one of the vomit bowls and waft me with it.' There was a silence for a moment, and then Sheila's face briefly appeared from under the curtain.

'It's not all about you, Pippa,' she admonished curtly with a grin, and dropped the drapes again. It was so unexpected I felt like laughing, but this really wasn't the time or place! Clearly unmoved by my plight, Sheila carried on assisting the consultant, and a few minutes later I felt him scooping the baby's head safely off my hand. Thank God! The baby seemed perfectly healthy, and it was a relief to be able to get my hand back, but it was the first cord prolapse I had experienced, and it was strange to say the least. We could have shaken hands in there!

Those waters can really take you by surprise. I was acting as the second midwife for one lady whose waters went as she was standing by the window of her room. Well, I have never seen so much amniotic fluid in my entire life! It was like a dam had broken and the entire room was flooded; at the same time, out slid the baby. Helen jumped up just in time to catch him, and then she slipped and slid across the room, trying to get the woman and her baby safely back to the bed. At one point I grabbed the baby just as I thought Helen might go tits up. It was all we could do to stay upright.

'I should have brought me cossie!' I joked, as I skidded across the floor. We were all laughing and joking about it, but it really was like sloshing through a shallow pond. Afterwards both Helen and I had to change our dresses, as we were soaked from head to toe.

We get into all sorts of funny positions to deliver babies. I've been on the floor, in the pool, squatting, on the bed –

you name it, I've been there. And we frequently end up covered in waters, blood, urine and meconium. Usually, it's fairly benign, and just a question of jumping in the shower, washing it off and changing into some clean scrubs, but that's not always the case. There are a few, rare occasions when we are exposed to real personal jeopardy. One time I was acting as second midwife at the point of delivery and, while the first midwife dealt with the mum and baby, it was my job to assist the dad with cutting the cord.

Usually, this is a really nice job, and a great way for the dad to get involved. I clamped the cord at both ends and showed him where to cut. He made the incision with cord scissors and straight away hit a blood vessel, which squirted all over my face. Blood ran down my face and neck and onto my arms, but worse, it was in my eyes. I tried to open them but all I could see was a dark crimson film.

'Helen, I can't open my eyes,' I said quietly and calmly, though inside I was horrified. 'Sorry, but I've got to go.'

'Okay,' she said, sensing my growing alarm. 'Let me just help you out here.' She took me by the shoulders and carefully manoeuvred me out of the door, my eyes still firmly shut.

'Don't worry,' I sang out to the family as I left. 'These things happen. It's now my time to go!' I didn't want them to feel guilty for what had happened – it wasn't their fault.

As soon I got into the corridor, I called out: 'Help! Need some help here, please!' I had no idea who was there because I had my eyes closed but, a few seconds later, I heard a voice next to me and felt a comforting hand on my shoulder.

'Pippa? Are you okay? What happened?' I recognised the Spanish accent of Marie, one of our ODPs (Operating Department Practitioner).

'Cord vessel erupted in my face,' I replied.

'Right, let's get you washed up and then we'll see where we're at.'

Marie steered me over to the staff bathroom, where we cleaned up my face and she gave me an eyewash.

'I think you better go straight down to A&E,' she said, as she washed the blood from my eyes and my vision gradually returned. She was right – technically, this was classed as a 'sharps injury'. Any 'sharps injury' where your skin is broken by a needle or sharp object – or 'needle stick', as they're sometimes known – demands an immediate blood test for HIV and other blood-borne diseases.

Reluctantly, I trudged off to A&E. I didn't feel too worried, because I had looked through the woman's hospital notes during the birth, so I knew she had tested negative for HIV. The chances were very slim that I could get HIV. But then the questions and doubts started to creep in. She'd had the test nine months previously, when she had first fallen pregnant. Who knew what she might have done since then?

I tried to stay calm and rational, thinking of the most likely outcome, as the A&E nurse took my bloods for testing – but it didn't help when I was sent off to see the Occupational Health Practitioner.

'You're at risk of HIV, Hep B, Hep C, syphilis, malaria, brucellosis and viral haemorrhagic fevers.' She reeled off the list as if giving me her weekly Tesco shopping order.

'As you're aware, we always have to err on the side of caution in cases like this. Your first HIV test will be back within a week, but then you'll have another in three months and a third three months after that. In the meantime, we strongly advise that you do not have unprotected sex with your partner, just in case there is a small chance you have contracted HIV. But don't worry – we have plenty of condoms we can supply you with.'

Good lord. I'd been pretty level-headed until then, but far from being reassuring, the OHP's little speech had the opposite effect. By the time I fell out of her office, bag of condoms in hand, I was a jangle of nerves. It was just as well Will and I were having a break from trying to make babies while we sorted out our new house.*

By now, we'd been together eighteen months, and though things were moving fast, it all felt right. Everything was falling into place. The day we got the keys of our new home, Will and I were so excited we wandered from room to room in a daze, saying to each other: 'It's ours. It's really ours!' The bed, sofas, table and chairs were all due to be delivered later that week, but we couldn't wait one more day to start living in our new house. We made up a small camp bed in the living room and we slept on that for the first week, camping out in our new home. It was blissful. For the first time we had our own space and could come and go as we pleased. We celebrated by getting a dog!

Still, Mum's disapproval gnawed at me. When I told her about our new Labradoodle puppy – a cross between a

---

* It would be nice if that was my one and only sharps injury but I've had two more since then, and both within a very short period of time. On the first occasion I was giving an injection to a lady and, just as I was putting the needle into the sharps box, I caught myself. The other incident happened a few weeks later. A woman had just given birth on the floor and my colleague was next to her, administering the oxytocin injection to help her deliver her placenta. As she stood up to put the needle in the sharps bin, she caught my leg. So that meant six more months of HIV tests and protected sex! Thank God the needles have changed now. After you've injected them, there's a flip that clips over and covers the needle so you can't get a needle stick. So hopefully that's the end of needle sticks for me, but that's not to say I won't get another squirt of blood in the eye!

Labrador and a Poodle – she seemed uninterested: 'I'm sure you know what you're doing, love. It's *your* life.'

It confused me. Mum had always been my biggest cheerleader, and I just couldn't understand this new disdain and negativity she had for me. When I relayed this all to Will, he sat and thought about it for a minute.

'Maybe she feels left out,' he said. 'I mean, from all those things she says to you, it sounds like she's resentful of *me*.'

'Don't be ridiculous!' I scoffed. 'Why would she be?'

'Think about it – with Rob, she had been really involved. He was round your house every night and she was cooking for him like he was her son. That's why you found it so difficult to leave him. He was like family. Now we're going off together and making all these big decisions without her. It's like she's losing her little girl.'

Maybe he had a point.

* * *

I was now twenty-five, gaining experience and confidence on the ward all the time. The further on you get in midwifery, the more you come across different conditions and complications. I'd noticed, for instance, that we tended to see a huge influx of women with pre-eclampsia in the spring, when the daffodils came out. And though pre-eclampsia is not uncommon, it is still a very high-risk condition, so we have to test all our women for the symptoms of high blood pressure, swelling and protein in the urine. If a woman is diagnosed with pre-eclampsia, she is given anti-hypertensive medication to lower the blood pressure and keep it at a stable rate, but we have to constantly assess the situation, to see if we need to get the baby delivered. High blood pressure is very dangerous for a baby. It can lead to abruption, which is when the placenta is pushed away from the uterine wall. If they abrupt then the baby can bleed out in utero. So any woman that presents with pre-eclampsia is admitted to the antenatal ward, so we can check their blood pressure every four hours.

If we don't deal with it, pre-eclampsia develops into eclampsia. That's when the mother starts to fit and we need to get them delivered straight away. No one is quite sure what causes eclampsia, but it is thought to be something to do with abnormal blood vessels formed in the placenta. Then, when that baby is born, everything subsides. But it is potentially life-threatening and anybody can get it. My close friend had it at twenty-five weeks with her first baby, and delivered at thirty weeks. And with her second baby, she had it again at twenty-eight weeks, and the baby was born at thirty-three weeks. She had to be given magnesium sulphate to stop her from fitting, but once she was started on that they had to get the baby delivered within forty-eight hours because it's not good for the baby.

Other conditions we have to watch out for include cholestasis, which is an increase in bile acids in the blood, causing a woman to itch on her hands, feet and abdomen. This is also a potentially life-threatening condition because the acid in the blood can cause the baby to go into cardiac arrest, leading to stillbirth. So, women suffering from cholestasis are usually induced at thirty-eight weeks, if they've not already gone into labour. We have to be so careful, because even the most innocent-sounding conditions can be very serious when you're pregnant. A simple urine infection, for example, can bring on early labour, as I was soon to discover.

* * *

It was eight months after we'd moved into our new home that I started to feel strange. My boobs hurt, and although I couldn't quite put my finger on it, I didn't feel exactly myself. When my period failed to show up, I decided to do a pregnancy test but it turned out negative. *Oh well,* I thought. *Must be a false alarm.* A week later, Will and I went out to a friend's birthday party and had a few drinks, but the next day I was dizzy, had a shocking headache and couldn't stop throwing up.

'This is more than just a hangover,' I said to Will. 'I think you better go to Asda and get me a pregnancy test.'

Will wasn't taking any chances – he came back with a whole selection of different tests.

'I only needed the one!' I laughed.

'If you're going to do something properly . . .' he said.

I peed on several assorted sticks and wands and we waited nervously for the results. I didn't have the heart to look myself so, after the full two minutes had passed, I told Will to go to the bathroom to get the tests. He returned seconds later, his face beaming with joy.

'Two red lines. Positive!' he shouted triumphantly, brandishing one of the pregnancy tests.

Then he held up another one: 'Positive!' And the third and fourth had the same result. Well, there was absolutely no doubt about it this time – I was definitely pregnant again.

11

Trust

'Please get back on the bed, Gemma,' I said as sweetly as I could.

'I can't. I just can't. I'm in bloody *agony*!' Gemma wailed, crouching in the corner, one hand on the wall, the other over her belly. I went over to her and knelt by her side, my hand on her shoulder.

'But if you get on the bed, we can monitor your baby,' I explained gently.

'*Urgghgh*,' she exhaled, now closing her eyes against the pain. I'm sure she couldn't hear me any more as the torment swept away all her senses. Right now, she was focused entirely on fighting the torture inside. Sam and I exchanged worried looks. Gemma had come in earlier in that day with a urine infection. She was only thirty-four weeks pregnant, but at that stage a urine infection can put a woman into early labour. So we had started her on antibiotics and kept her in for monitoring. As the day wore on, Gemma started complaining of pains she felt sure were contractions, and she was now showing all the signs of labouring.

Sam and I slid quietly out of the room together. Officially, Gemma was under Sam's care that day, but she'd called me in to try to persuade Gemma to stay on the bed. It was a very tricky situation.

'If she won't keep the monitor on her, we've *got* to get the registrar to look her over,' she said, sighing. It was about the fourth time she had said that to me in the past two hours. The problem was we had asked the registrar to attend several times already and she had refused. The last time I'd asked, she had exploded at me: 'Pippa, I have seen that lady already and she is *not* in labour.'

'Yes, I know. But we think the situation may have changed since you last saw her.'

'Not that quickly. Look, I'm extremely busy. Later, okay?'

I went back to Sam, and she knew from my expression I had been sent away with a flea in my ear.

'I'm sure she's in labour,' she muttered.

The problem was we weren't allowed to examine her to find out for certain. NHS guidelines state that a woman has to be full term – i.e. over thirty-seven weeks – for a midwife to examine her. Given that Gemma was still only thirty-four weeks, she needed a full review by a doctor. It was so infuriating. Every single one of us midwives would have been able to tell in a few seconds if Gemma was in labour from a quick assessment of her cervix with our fingers. I'm probably more qualified at doing this than most doctors! You get very used to judging the dilation just by the feel of the cervix. Of course, it can vary slightly, according to who is doing the examining, but not too much. Maybe a centimetre either side. Normally, when a lady comes in who is full term, we'll examine her, see how far along she is and, if she looks like she's in labour, we'll spend some time with her, seeing how frequent the contractions are, how strong they seem and how well they're coping. We'll find out what pain relief they've taken at home already and make an assessment of whether we need to examine them or not. But if someone is preterm like Gemma we don't go in with an examination straight away because our fingers can stimulate the cervix, causing it to dilate, bringing on labour. The registrar had seen Gemma when she'd first come in, but she had not assessed her in the past four hours, and now Sam and the LWC were both getting worried. And they'd called me over for 'back up' when Gemma came off the monitor.

'I just don't know what to do,' Sam whispered, as we stood outside the door. 'I think she's having contractions, I really do. We need to try and keep her on the monitor.'

At that point, the door opened, and Gemma's red sweating face appeared.

'I'm going out for a fag,' she puffed.

'Gemma, I really don't think that's a good idea,' said Sam.

'I need a fucking fag!' Gemma snapped. 'It hurts, okay? You can't give me anything and I need something to take the edge off.'

'But if you stay on the monitor . . .'

'Fuck that! Give me an epidural and I'll stay on the bed for the rest of the night! But if you won't give me anything for the pain, I can't just lie around in agony. It hurts. Right?' Gemma jostled us out of the way with her considerable frame and waddled down the corridor.

Sam and I watched helplessly, and I heard real despair in Sam's voice as she whispered, 'What am I meant to do?'

There was nothing we could do to stop her – and nothing more we could give her for her pain because officially she wasn't in labour. She'd had the recommended dose of paracetamol and that was it. She didn't get on with the Tens machine, had no time for the aromatherapy oils, and she had shunned a hot bath. We couldn't offer her any more than that because, according to the registrar, she *wasn't in labour*.

'Right.' Jen had been watching this scene unfold from the nurses' station. 'Sam, you get back to the registrar and you ask her to attend again.'

'Again?'

'Yes. And again and again until she bloody well comes!'

* * *

It was a gruelling night. Gemma was up and down like a jack-in-the-box, and as often as Sam asked for the registrar to review her, she kept getting knock-backs. She was busy, it seemed – at first with C-sections and then a forceps delivery. And though I could understand that certain emergencies came first, I had begun to feel it was becoming a battle of wills rather than a genuine response to a medical request. The registrar had dug her heels in, pulled rank and decided she was not going to see Gemma.

Finally, at 11 p.m., she was free to attend. By then, Gemma was beside herself, screaming in agony. She had completely lost it – she was on and off the bed, in and out of her clothes, in and out of the hospital, taking herself off for a smoke. Her partner and mother were doing their best to keep her calm, but it was an impossible task. We just couldn't keep her on the monitor, and when we did have her on the bed, the fact that she was a large lady with a raised BMI meant it wasn't always easy to find the foetal heartbeat.

Most of the night, I had my own lady to deal with, but every now and then I'd bump into Sam in the corridor, looking increasingly stressed. The next thing I knew, Gemma was being wheeled off down the corridor to the labour ward and Sam called out to me: 'Seven centimetres! She's seven centimetres dilated!'

I went back into the room with my lady but, then, about ten minutes later, I heard the emergency buzzer go. I raced out to see the light going over Gemma's room. Several others had also responded to the buzzer, and together we piled into the room. It looked like Gemma was just about to deliver into Sam's arms, but the expression on Sam's face said it all. She was pale and fearful.

'Lost the foetal heartbeat during the transfer,' the registrar explained. 'Someone get me the scanner for foetal heart rate abdominally.'

It was only a matter of a few more minutes before Gemma delivered her baby, and straight away the little girl was transferred to me and the paediatricians for resuscitation. She was pale and floppy. We started by giving five long inflation breaths, trying to ensure a chest rise, which would mean we were getting oxygen into the baby. But the chest didn't rise, so we repositioned the head to open the airway. Then we started chest compressions.

'Check time, please,' said the paediatrician.

'Baby born at twenty-three fifty-seven.'

'Okay, so how old are we now?'

'Two minutes old, the timer is on.'

'Can you have another listen to heartbeat, please?'

'Heartbeat less than one hundred.'

'Open neonatal resus trolley so we can intubate.'

Sam was now kneeling next to Gemma, helping to deliver the placenta and doing her best to reassure her.

'The paediatricians have her now,' she was saying softly. 'They're doing their best.'

'Is she okay?' Gemma asked tearfully. 'I can't hear her crying. Why isn't she crying? Is she okay?'

We worked on that baby for forty-five heartbreaking minutes. It was awful – the whole time I was giving cardiac massage to this child I could hear Gemma's sobs behind me. But it was no good. The baby never got a heartbeat; she never moved or took a breath. There were no signs of life and, eventually, the consultant called the time of death.

I walked out of the room and was immediately overcome with despair. You try your best but sometimes it's not enough. I leaned back against the wall and sobbed, the healthcare nurse put her arm around me, and we wept together. Then the senior house officer broke down. And the paediatric consultant. In fact, every single member of staff who had been in that room cried for the baby we couldn't save. Well, all except one – the registrar didn't shed a tear or show any emotion at all; there was no sign of remorse or regret.

No matter how many times I've experienced it, I never get used to losing a baby. And all of us involved in that tragic birth experienced that same terrible helplessness and despair at not being able to save her. *Why? Why had this baby died? Could we have prevented it?* Of course, our feelings were nothing compared to the mother's, but you feel the loss deeply. I went home that night and sobbed my heart out.

By now, I was five months pregnant and things weren't exactly going well. Just like with my first pregnancy, I was bleeding on and off throughout, and it made me fear the worst. Mum knew all about it. I'd decided to tell her about the pregnancy straight away. Recalling how lonely I'd felt after the first miscarriage, I realised that if things didn't go well this time I would need her support. I should have guessed that she wasn't going to be overly thrilled by the news. Instead of congratulating me, she just nodded slowly before sounding a note of caution.

'Is this really what you want?' she asked, her brow furrowed, her head tilted to one side. 'I mean, you haven't known Will all that long. A baby is a really big thing. You'll be tied to each other for life.'

'Of course it's what I want, Mum,' I insisted, laughing. 'It's what we both want – to have our own family. We're really happy. I just wish you could see that.'

'Hmm . . . we'll see.'

'Mum, this is going to be *your grandchild*. Whether you like Will or not, whether you approve of him or not, I would really appreciate it if you could get on board with this.'

She nodded curtly and walked out of the room. I sighed. Why was it so hard for her to accept my choices?

But the longer the pregnancy went on, the more Mum came round to the idea. I invited her along to the twelve-week scan, and she came to the next scan, too. Each time, the scans showed that everything was normal and, this time around, my pregnancy hormones were at the right levels. Nevertheless, I continued to bleed, and I couldn't relax and enjoy being pregnant because in the back of my mind I was just waiting to miscarry. One time I was seated on the bed, talking to a lady in labour, when I felt a 'popping' sensation down below. By the time I stood up I had bled right through my knickers, my uniform and onto the bedsheets. I was mortified and took myself straight down the corridor to Triage for assessment.

They had a look inside me using a speculum but could see no obvious reason for the bleed – everything was normal, the placenta wasn't too low and they couldn't tell where the bleeding might be coming from. Even so, they decided to keep me in for monitoring for the next twelve hours, just in case it happened again. I went from colleague to patient in ten minutes flat. I suppose there are times when it's helpful to work on a labour ward!

I tried, but I couldn't ignore the bleeds. They made me wary of getting too attached to the baby growing inside me, just in case the pregnancy didn't go to full term. In my head, I set myself little goals: *if I can get to twelve weeks, then I'll be okay.* But then, after twelve weeks, I found I still couldn't relax, so I set myself another goal, to get to sixteen weeks. *When I get to sixteen weeks I'll relax and enjoy it.* And yet, when I hit sixteen weeks, it was the same again. This went on the whole way through the pregnancy.

I was off work the week after Gemma's baby died. I'd had another bleed and the doctor encouraged me to rest as much as possible. Fortunately, the senior team were really good about giving me the time off that I needed. I suppose, given that we were a labour ward, it was the least they could do, but it added up to quite a lot of time off the ward. It was one week on, one week off; one week on, one week off the whole way – and I wasn't used to sitting about all day.

Will was keen for me to slow down. Every time I got up to put a wash on or clear the plates, he'd yell at me to 'sit down and put your bloody feet up!'

'It's not that easy,' I sulked. 'I like to be busy. It doesn't suit me just lying around doing nothing all day.'

'Some women would die for the chance to laze around the whole time with a partner willing to do all the cooking and clearing up.'

'Not if they'd seen the way *you* clean up.'

'Are you complaining?'

'You do know you have to use hot water *and* washing-up liquid to clean the dishes.'

'Oh, you cheeky cow!'

That was just how Will and I were with each other, always joking and ribbing each other. Neither of us liked confrontation – it wasn't in my nature or his.

* * *

During one of those weeks where I was able to be at work, Sam and I were on the same nightshift and she filled me in on the situation with Gemma.

'She's put in a complaint,' she said. 'I don't blame her. I mean, if the registrar had reviewed her earlier we could have done something. But we wasted so much time – *hours* - when she could have been given proper pain relief and we'd have been able to keep her on the monitor.'

Sam felt angry and let down at what happened during Gemma's birth, but she felt sure the subsequent investigation would bring to light the failings of the senior team. After all, the words 'registrar asked to review' were scrawled all over Gemma's notes.

'Do you think she'll be disciplined?' I asked Sam.

'I really hope so. I mean, God forbid that happens to another lady. If we don't learn our lesson this time, it'll just happen again.'

Six months later, the investigation concluded and, as expected, the hospital admitted negligence. But instead of laying the blame with the registrar, they'd somehow managed to blame the midwives! The senior management team claimed that we had not done enough to get the registrar to attend. I was shocked at the conclusion. It was written all over the notes that we had done everything in our power to bring a doctor into the room. It was all there in black and white – and yet somehow the blame had been put back onto us. I was astonished that the registrar had managed to wriggle out of taking responsibility for her failure to attend. Sam wept floods of angry tears when we read the hospital report.

'They've stabbed us in the back,' she said. 'How could they do that? How?'

We had been betrayed by the hospital management. At the moment we had expected them to tell the truth they had hung us out to dry. It shook me up quite badly to see that report. To my mind, the whole ward worked on trust. Our birthing mothers put their trust in us, and likewise we trusted our colleagues to be there when we needed them. And if they weren't, then they had to own up to their mistakes. This was a slap in the face. For the first time, I felt the trust between us and our managers had been broken – and that made me feel vulnerable and exposed.

12

Breathe . . .

What was that? I shot out of the bath. It felt like something had popped inside me. I dried myself off, trying to waft away the smell of clary sage, then pulled a towel around my gigantic bump and waddled to the landing. It was 5.30 p.m. and, though I was just a couple of days past my due date, I was desperate for my little girl to come. I had been on maternity leave for two weeks already, and now that the baby room was painted and we'd bought everything we needed for our first few months as parents, I was impatient to meet my daughter. We knew it was a little girl from the second scan. The sonographer had passed the ultrasound over my bump and straightaway I could tell. I shot Will an excited look and he said: 'You know, don't you?'

'It's a baby girl!' I squealed. 'We're having a little girl!'

All day long I'd been experiencing little niggles and pains, but nothing approaching a contraction, so I'd decided to have a go at all those things they tell you to do to bring on labour. Earlier in the day, I'd taken our dog, Biscuit, out for a long walk and I'd been drinking raspberry leaf tea like it was going out of fashion. Will had strict instructions to make us a hot curry for our tea and, in the meantime, I decided to take a bath using clary sage, an aromatherapy oil thought to bring on contractions. On the labour ward we never recommend using more than a few drops in the bath, but I was sceptical that a few drops would be effective so, in a moment of pure madness, I poured in half the bottle.

'Will!' I called out from the landing. He was in the kitchen, preparing our dinner.

'Will!' I called again. 'Wi- Oh!' A huge gush of water poured out of me and onto the carpet.

'Oh my God, oh my God! WILL!' I screamed.

'What? What is it?' He appeared at the bottom of the stairs.

'I think my waters have gone, Look! My waters have gone.'

'Bloody hell!' Will saw me standing in the middle of the rapidly spreading wet patch. At the same instant, I felt a huge swell of pain growing in my belly, getting stronger and more intense by the second. I was completely taken aback by the strength of the contraction, and crouched down, doubled over in agony. *Too much clary sage. I've used too much bloody clary sage!* When the contraction had passed, Will walked me downstairs to the living room, but in another thirty seconds I was overcome by yet another.

'Oh my God . . . oh my God . . . oh my God.' I breathed hard, completely overcome by the intensity of the contraction. *What happened to a contraction every two minutes?* I thought they were supposed to build slowly over a number of hours. I'd gone from nought to agony in thirty seconds flat! 'Get the Tens machine, Will! The Tens machine! Oh . . . ow . . . *ngggg* . . . too much clary sage.'

Will dashed off to get the machine, opening all the windows in the house, trying to get rid of the smell of clary sage. *How do women do this?* I wondered, suddenly in awe of every single birthing mother I'd assisted. *It's not meant to hurt this much, surely!*

Will returned a minute later with the handheld device and strapped the pads onto my back. We switched the machine on – it's meant to help with pain management by emitting small electric currents, but it took just one contraction to convince me that it wasn't going to touch my pain.

'Oh, it's useless! I can't deal with this,' I exclaimed, ripping the pads from my back, and, with that, I picked up the phone and called the ward. Bev answered.

'It's started and it's just too much,' I told her. 'I can't cope. I'm coming in.'

* * *

On the ward, Bev, Sam and Helen were all there to greet me – ah, my second family! I was instantly reassured by their presence. Bev had insisted she would be my midwife for the birth – I think she would have fought off a herd of angry baboons for the privilege – and when we'd chatted about it over a cup of tea in the staffroom a few months previously I had been deliberately vague.

'I'm not doing a birthing plan,' I'd said. 'I've seen too many birthing plans go wrong. We'll just have to see what happens . . . take it as it comes.'

'Yeah, but if you had a choice?'

'Well, if I had a choice, I wouldn't mind a pool birth.' Now I begged her for an epidural.

'What happened to the pool birth?' she asked, a mischievous

smile on her lips. *Goddamn Beverley. What a fool I'd been to tell her what I wanted!*

'No, no, no, forget the pool birth. No pool. I'm a midwife and I know I need a fucking epidural, and I need it quickly,' I insisted. 'Blame the clary sage, blame Will's penis, blame . . . *arrhhhhhh*, please! I'm begging, get me an epidural!'

'Well, let's have a look at you first and then we'll see where we're at.' But when Bev examined me, she found I was only 2 cms dilated.

Only 2 cms? I was beside myself. *How can I stand any more of this?*

'And judging by the suture lines on baby's head, she is lying occiput posterior,' she went on. 'So, this might take some time. Why don't you go home and come back in a little while?'

Oh no. Back to back. That meant my baby's back was against mine and she was facing forward. Normally, the baby's head faces the bottom and this is the easiest way for them to deliver due to the dimensions of their skulls. If she's back to back, she still has to rotate 180 degrees before delivery.

That's when I panicked. *First baby? Back to back? I'm going to theatre – I just know it.*

'God, no. I'm not going home. I'm going to end up in theatre, aren't I? Dear God! Seriously, Bev, I'm a midwife and I know it's not meant to hurt this much.'

'Yes it is.'

'Oh shut up! Please, please, please, just give me an epidural.'

'I tell you what, let's just start you on some diamorphine, yeah?'

'Yes – anything! But be quick about it!'

Breathe . . .

She returned a few minutes later with the injection and my whole body was flooded with relief when the painkiller finally kicked in, taking the edge off the contractions enough for me to relax a little. Will, meanwhile, was enjoying himself, playing with the stereo in our room. He'd been through all the 'ambient' CDs – the chirping crickets, rainforest noises, birdsong and beach waves, and now he'd moved onto marine mammals.

'Get that fucking whale song off the radio now,' I groaned. 'I listen to that shit every day!'

'Well, what do you want to do?' he asked meekly.

'I don't know. Why don't you put a film on the laptop? Something easy, something gentle.' He started scrolling through our Netflix account.

'How about *Schindler's List*?' he asked, deadpan.

'Ha ha,' I replied sarcastically. My boyfriend thinks he's a bloody comedian!

For the next two hours, I dozed as Will watched a Michael McIntyre show on the laptop, perched on the food tray next to the bed. Every now and then a contraction woke me up and I'd come round to the sound of Will laughing his head off. Meanwhile, I was convinced we were still in the middle of a conversation we'd started twenty minutes earlier.

'So, we'll move the chest of drawers to the kitchen then,' I mumbled sleepily to him.

'Hmmm? What's that?' Will replied, eyes fixed to the screen.

'With the lounge . . . we'll paint it grey. And we'll move the drawers,' I drawled incoherently, before closing my eyes and dropping off again. This went on for the next two hours, until Bev came back in and examined me again.

'Four centimetres,' she said. 'Getting there.'

'Please, *please* put me in the pool now,' I begged, the effects of the diamorphine starting to wear off.

'It's a little early,' she said hesitantly.

'Oh please, Bev! I need to get in there now. I really do.'

'It's just too early, darling.'

'Okay, give me another diamorphine injection then. Something – I need *something*!'

Bev shook her head: 'You know as well as I do that if I give you another injection then we can't give you a pool birth.'

'I don't care. I don't want a sodding pool birth. I just want the pain to go away.'

'I'll tell you what we'll do. We'll get you over to the pool room, all right?'

'Okay, okay,' I puffed, too distracted by the pain to argue.

'In the meantime, why don't you have something to eat?' Bev suggested. 'We need to keep your energy levels up.'

I sent Will off to Burger King, as I had a real craving for chicken nuggets and a strawberry milkshake. But the moment he arrived back with the food, the smell made me want to retch. Ten minutes later, I was cramming it into my mouth.

'You're all over the shop,' he said, grinning at me.

'No I'm not.'

'Honestly, you don't know if you're coming or going. It's quite funny, really. It's bloody fantastic that I never have to do this. I really appreciate not having a vagina today! By the way, your mum's here, I saw her at Reception. Do you want to see her?'

'Yeah, send her in.'

Breathe . . .

My mum! I need my mum. I'm desperate to see my mum.
She gave me a big hug when she arrived – and promptly
told me off.

'I don't know why you took the diamorphine,' she tutted
disapprovingly.

*Oh, for goodness sake! I can't bear to be around you if
you're going to be like this.*

'Yes, well, anyway, you have to leave now, Mum. I'm going
to the pool.'

'But I've only just this second got here!'

'Yes, but I'm going to another room now, so off you go.' By
now the drugs had worn off completely and I was back to
square one, doubled up in agony, no idea or mental strength
to know what I was saying or doing, the pain engulfing me
and all my senses, from thought to reasoning. To my mind,
I was probably going to end up in theatre in the early hours,
so it was best if Mum went home now anyway. She would
need all her energy for later.

'Come on,' Bev said. 'Let's get you to the pool room.'

In the time it took for me to get from one room to another,
I lost the plot completely.

'I need a shower!' I yelled, and threw off all my clothes,
door wide open, in full view of everyone and anyone in
the corridor.

'Hi, Sheila!' I waved to Sheila, who trotted past and gave
me a cheery wave back: 'Hiya, Pippa, love.' I got into the
shower and seconds later I was out again.

'Gas and air!' I yelled at Will. He handed me the inhaler
and I took in three long, deep puffs.

'No, it's not doing anything,' I complained. Now I leaned
over the edge of the pool, which was at waist height, and

begged him to rub my back. But the moment he put his hands on me, I shrieked: 'Argh! Get off. Don't touch me.'

The pain was so intense I was completely swamped by it. It was like being swept up in a tsunami of agony that overtook my mind and all my senses, so much so I couldn't tell what I was doing any more. At one point, I was shouting, 'My clitoris! My clitoris!' Then I stood there, with the portable canister in hand, leaning over the pool, completely naked, taking in long gasps of gas and air through each contraction. And that's when it got serious.

'Pippa, what are you doing?' Will asked.

'Nothing,' I muttered. 'I just need the gas.'

'No seriously, Pippa. What are you *doing*?'

'What do you mean?'

Suddenly I realised what he was talking about – I felt myself bearing down.

'Oh no. I think I'm *pushing*! I can't, it's too soon. I just need an epidural.'

Will pulled the buzzer and Jen burst in just as another contraction started. 'Are you alright, Pippa? Pippa! What are you doing?'

'I'm pushing!'

'Let me have a quick look.' She got on her knees and bent down to check, then stood up pretty sharpish. 'Okay, let's get this pool run!' she said.

Jen started running the water, and Bev raced in just in time to see me getting in the pool – it was only a few inches deep at this point but I didn't care.

'Call my mum,' I whispered to Will. 'I want her back here.'

'Are you sure?'

'Yeah, yeah,' I said, and smiled. I knew the baby was

coming and, despite everything that had happened between us, she was still my mum and I wanted her by my side. The water kept running and I now felt myself pushing properly. Will took hold of my hand and Bev watched in awe at how well I was doing, just occasionally listening to our baby's heartbeat. Mum was back in the room for the last ten minutes and, at 11.11 p.m., my little girl was born and I pulled her straight up onto my chest.

'Is she alright?' I asked Bev, who was at my shoulder.

'Yeah, she's beautiful.' She smiled at me through her tears.

Will too had tears in his eyes. 'You did it,' he said quietly. 'Well done.'

'I did it!' I wept.

We named her Betty and she was absolutely gorgeous. I was so grateful to Bev afterwards – she knew what I wanted and she made sure I got it, no matter how much I had begged for an epidural.

'You were a nightmare!' Will laughed later when he recounted the whole five hours of labour. 'And I wouldn't have missed it for the world.'

My birthing experience had given me a whole new respect for the women who came onto the ward and the pain they were experiencing. I now knew what they meant when they told me they were in agony. Luckily, Betty latched onto my breast straightaway, and after the first twenty-four hours we were allowed to go home. I loved being a mum from the start. Despite the sleeplessness, I was in a lovely little bubble with Betty and would have happily stayed that way – if she hadn't got ill.

It was ten days after the birth and Will had just taken her out in the pram for a few hours to give me some rest. When she came back, there was something about her that didn't look quite right. She had a vacant stare, as if she was looking straight through me. Then, when I put her to the breast, she refused to feed.

'Something's not right,' I said to Will, but I couldn't for the life of me work out what it was. I kept doing her observations but they all came back normal. The only thing was, she wouldn't feed. I called the ward several times, but they reassured me: 'She's fine, Pippa. If she's sleeping, make the most of it, get some sleep yourself.' Only I didn't feel reassured. I knew how hard it was to make telephone assessments of babies without seeing them, and something gnawed at me deep inside. Are they right? Is she okay? Maybe if they were looking at her, they would see what I was seeing.

All night long, I worried over her, wondering whether to take her into hospital. Then, at around 1 a.m., I tried a cup feed to get some milk into her. By this point she'd not fed for nine hours and I didn't want her blood sugars to drop too low. That's when she stopped breathing and went white and floppy in my arms. She was completely unresponsive.

No time to panic. At that moment, my midwife training kicked in. I was on autopilot. I grabbed a towel and started rubbing her, trying to stimulate her tiny body. She started breathing again and her tone and colour came back. But I wasn't taking any chances. We needed to get to hospital and fast. Will called the ambulance, but they were coming from a fair distance and they didn't get to us for another twenty minutes.

Betty stopped breathing again before the ambulance arrived, and this time the towel didn't work straight away, so I had to do compressions on her tiny chest to keep her breathing, blowing over her mouth and nose to get air into her. After a few compressions, I put my ear to her chest to listen for a heartbeat. I needed a stethoscope but I didn't have any equipment at home. Meanwhile, Will was on the phone to 999, begging them to hurry up.

'Come on! Please can you get someone here NOW! For God's sake, where are they?' he yelled. Finally, after what felt like a lifetime, the paramedics arrived, and Betty was blue-lighted to hospital. She stopped breathing twice more in the ambulance before we arrived, and then she was rushed onto the neonatal care unit. Until then, I had stayed calm and composed, just dealing with the situation in the same way I'd deal with any emergency on the ward. But the moment she was taken off my hands by the paediatric team, placed on a little resus trolley, smothered by busy hands that were attaching her to snaking wires and tubes, it hit me all at once. This was my baby! And this was the most terrifying experience of my life. I started to shake violently and then collapsed in tears.

'We nearly lost her!' I gasped, my body racked by great juddering sobs. I was beside myself, unable to stop crying. 'I knew something wasn't right. Why didn't I go with my instincts? We should have brought her in sooner.'

'You saved her life!' Will said, shaking his head in wonder. 'Don't beat yourself up, Pip. You did everything right.'

In the neonatal unit, Betty was wired to what looked like countless machines and given a battery of tests, including a lumbar puncture to test for infections of the spine and brain. That was horrendous. Will couldn't even watch, but I held her the whole time. I simply couldn't let her out of my sight.

And even though I've held babies for lumbar punctures before, there's nothing like that ear-splitting cry when the huge needle is first inserted into their spine. Hearing it from your own child is even more heart-rending. I was a mess, breaking down in tears all the time. In the end, the doctors found Betty had an infection, a heart murmur and a virus all at once – her poor little body just couldn't cope and had shut down. She looked so helpless lying there, a mass of wires, tubes and drips, as the doctors tried to stabilise her. I was just so grateful that she was being treated at the hospital where I worked – the paediatric staff and doctors were all amazing. I couldn't fault them for a second.

* * *

Once Betty was stable, I called my mum and dad to tell them what had happened and they rushed to hospital to see us. It wasn't until the following day, while Mum was watching Betty, I took a minute to pop across to the labour ward to tell my colleagues what had happened overnight. At first, they almost failed to recognise me, as I was in such a state – my hair was a mess, I was horribly sleep-deprived and still wearing my pyjamas from the night before. They could see what a state I was in, and they put their arms around me as I poured my heart out to them, telling them what had happened and how horrendous it had been. From that moment, they all took it in turns to come over to see me in the neonatal unit.

All in all, we were in hospital for a week together, and I didn't leave Betty's side the whole time. I slept in a recliner chair by her bedside, watching her, making sure she was okay. Betty was so poorly she slept almost that entire time, just trying to fight off the infection. Will was working fifteen-hour shifts, grabbing something to eat, coming in to see us then going home and doing it all again the next day. It was a testing time for all of us.

'Come on, darling, you have to have something to eat,' insisted the sandwich lady when she visited our room.

'No, honestly, I'm fine,' I yawned, stretching my legs out. It had been another rough night. I found it so difficult to sleep in that damn chair – even so, it didn't cross my mind for a second to go home.

'You're feeding, my darling, you need to keep your strength up.'

'Yeah, okay.' I smiled, picking out a tuna and cucumber roll from her trolley. Since Betty wasn't able to breastfeed, I was expressing in order to give her my milk through a bottle. I kept trying, but each time I put her to the breast, her oxygen levels dropped. She just couldn't drink and breathe at the same time.

When we finally got home, I carried on expressing because Betty would now only take milk through the bottle. It was tough going. At one point I got very bad mastitis from a blocked milk duct and ended up in utter agony. But I pushed on through. Like a lot of new mums, I was utterly determined to do everything 'right'. And in my mind that meant giving her breast milk, even if she wouldn't actually take it from my breast. I can't say I enjoyed being attached to the pump for hours on end – it made me feel like a Jersey cow – but I persisted nonetheless.

'Don't you think you've done enough?' Will asked one day, as I nursed a sore, swollen boob with a pack of frozen peas. I was still on antibiotics for the mastitis.

'It's the best thing for her,' I insisted.

'Really?' He seemed sceptical. 'I mean, I understand in the first few weeks it's got all those nutrients and things in, but now that she's five months old, she'll be absolutely fine on formula. Are you sure you're doing this for her or is it for you?'

'Her, of course!' I shot back indignantly. I knew Will only had my best interests at heart, but I was determined to do my best for Betty, even if it bloody killed me!

I was still expressing by the time I went back to work a year after giving birth. As the big day approached, I felt more and more anxious about returning to the ward after such a long break. Would I be able to remember all the things that had come naturally a year earlier? So much had happened. A lifetime had passed in the year I'd been away. Was I ready to go back? And, most worrying of all, how would I handle being away from Betty for up to fourteen hours at a time?

I loved being a mum, and Betty was my whole world. In our year together we had grown inseparable and I absolutely adored being around her 24/7, watching her grow and develop her own funny personality. She was a delight, and I had well and truly adapted to the 'mummy routine', caring for her every need, cleaning up, cooking and pumping in between. How could I bear to be away from her for so long? How could I possibly fit work into our new routine? My worries loomed larger every day.

13

Changes

'What on earth is *that*?' I pointed to a sign in the staff-room that had appeared during my maternity leave.

Angela rolled her eyes: 'I know. It's madness, isn't it?'

The sign said that midwives were now forbidden from taking tea, coffee or any hot drinks onto the ward. We were allowed to take in a water bottle with a 'sealable top', but that was it. Obviously, tea was some sort of safety hazard now! The management team had even installed a 'Hydration Station' – basically, a large water cooler – in the staff room, from which we could fill up our bottles, but alongside it there were a whole list of do's and don'ts. I started to read out the list from the sign: *Do not walk around with your drink. Water bottles are not to be taken into the clinical area. Do not wash your cup in a clinical area,* and *Do not use the hydration station as a social gathering area.*

'Eh? Does that mean we aren't allowed to talk to each other over the water cooler?'

'I know, I know.' Angela shook her head.

'Where are we meant to talk to each other, then?' This was unbelievable. Now we were explicitly being forbidden from chatting to each other at the 'hydration station'. Hadn't they heard of the phrase 'water cooler moment'? It is famously the place at work where people chat. Even worse was the unbearably patronising sign-off at the end: *Don't forget to put your patient's needs before your own!*

I sighed and sat down again. A lot had changed in the twelve months I'd been on maternity leave – a new management team had taken over and the walls of the staffroom were now plastered with various signs – lists of do's and don'ts, 'good practice' reminders and some outlining brand-new guidelines.

'Do they honestly want us to take care of a labouring woman for hours on end without even a cup of tea to sip on?' I asked Angela.

'They think it looks unprofessional,' Angela laughed. 'As if our women care!'

'So, let me get this straight,' I said. 'They say it's okay to sip from a water bottle but it looks unprofessional to sip from a mug?'

'I know! What's the difference? It's not like we have the time to get off the ward to make a cup of tea or get a coffee, so basically they're telling us we can't have a drink any more.'

'They haven't got a clue!'

'I wouldn't pay it much attention, Pippa.' Angela leaned in conspiratorially. 'I just ask my lady if she's happy for me to have a cuppa and then I bring in my tea anyway. It's like I always say – new faces, same old nonsense.'

I have to say, it wasn't the easiest transition back to work after maternity leave with Betty. I knew our hospital trust had come under increasing financial pressure in the last few years, but I wasn't aware of this having any serious impact on our ward until the new Band 8 management team was brought in. We never usually had contact with the Band 8s – Navy Blues, we called them, because of the colour of their uniform – as their offices were elsewhere on the hospital site. Our only contact was with the labour ward managers – Band 7s – who organised the shifts and rotas. Band 8s controlled budgets and staffing, and we barely saw them at all. Every now and again they sent out reminder emails to keep us all in line, like telling us not to eat on the ward. Getting caught munching at work meant an instant disciplinary, though it wasn't an issue on the ward at night when all the Band 8s had gone home.

Now the new management team had brought with them a whole raft of cost-saving measures. One of these was to change the method of clocking in and off the ward. In the past, each midwife would register the time she arrived and left the ward by swiping her badge on the door. In this way, management could keep an accurate record of how much overtime we had all done and pay us accordingly. But the badge method had been ditched, and now each of us needed to be signed off by a Band 7 or higher when we left for the day. And that worked fine if you did normal hours, but if I stayed to do overtime till late at night, my manager might have left before me. In which case, there would be nobody to verify my extra hours. So naturally the amount of overtime we all recorded – and were paid – went down. It was no reflection of the amount of overtime we had actually done, of course, just the fact that it wasn't recorded. The odd half hour or hour here and there . . . it all adds up.

Since the hospital was on an efficiency drive, we were no longer allowed to pay for agency staff to cover shifts when we were understaffed. And if staff left their jobs for whatever reason, the posts were left unfilled for months at a time due to lack of funding. This meant staff shortages had become the norm. On my very first day back after maternity leave, I was brought in to assist on a triplet C-section. I was astounded. I'd been off the ward for twelve months. I was completely out of practice and I hadn't even had a chance to catch up with all the new guidelines. I was rather hoping that in my first week I'd be able to ease myself back in with a few straightforward deliveries. Yet here I was assisting in a very rare and risky case of a triplet C-section at thirty-three weeks.

'Are you sure you want me in there?' I asked Laura, the Labour Ward Coordinator on duty. 'I haven't been in theatre for over a year.'

'I really don't have any choice,' she replied. 'I literally don't have anyone else.'

They had to muster as big a team as they could, just in case all three babies needed resuscitation, so there was no hiding away for me. Thankfully, everything went according to plan and the tiny babies were all born healthy and whisked off to the neonatal unit. It was such a relief, but that was a difficult first day back – no paddling in the shallows for me, I was hurled straight back in at the deep end.

There was a host of other new rules and guidelines with which I had to quickly bring myself up to speed, but the thing that affected me most was the new management's attitude towards me expressing for Betty. I had planned to keep her on the breast for the first eighteen months, but that idea gained little support among the management team on our ward. It all stemmed from the fact that we were now permanently short-staffed.

'Louise, can you get someone to cover me?' I asked the LWC five hours into one shift.

'Why?' she asked.

'I have to pump.'

'Erm . . . do you have to do it *now*?'

'Yes! I'm in agony. Seriously, I need to do this.' My breasts were so swollen with milk they were practically hard.

'Erm . . . can I get back to you in half an hour?' she said distractedly.

'Not really. Come on, Louise, I need to do this now or I'll end up leaking over this lovely lady in labour!' I tried to make a joke of it but inside I was seething. *We're midwives, for God's sake. Why are they making it so difficult for me to breastfeed?*

It wasn't the only time. In fact, I found it increasingly difficult to express at work because the management team made me feel like a massive inconvenience for even asking. I was just trying to do the right thing for my baby, and I was totally within my rights to take twenty minutes off every six hours to pump. But from the way they reacted you'd think I'd just asked to sleep with their husbands!

'Really? *Now*?' the LWCs would respond to my requests, flipping manically through their clipboards to see if they had any free hands to take over.

'Yes, now,' I'd reply, feeling guilty about leaving them in the lurch but also in physical discomfort from my overly full breasts. *Why was it always so difficult?* We actively promote the 'breast is best' approach, and yet I wasn't being given the time to do it. I knew it wasn't really the coordinator's fault – being so short-staffed, they were under so much pressure themselves and always did their best.

'I might have to jump in myself,' was often the reply. LWCs weren't meant to cover for us, but these days there was little alternative. Then, of course, I'd have to ask them twice in a twelve-hour shift.

'Again? So soon?'

'Well, it's either that or I pop home to feed her myself. Your choice!' I'd smile sweetly, but inside I was genuinely upset at being made to feel bad about what should have been a natural right. I didn't blame them, the Band 7s – it wasn't their fault we were understaffed. Whose fault was it? I felt like blaming the Band 8s, who seemed utterly against the idea of covering me properly for the time I needed to pump, but what financial pressures were they under? Whoever was to blame, the irony that a labour ward was an unsupportive environment for a breastfeeding mother was not lost on me.

One of the Navy Blues – a particularly strident woman called Lina, who had already given me a ticking off for wearing the wrong type of socks – even stopped me in the corridor one day to say, 'Oh, I hear you're not expressing any more, Pippa. That's good then,' before marching off again. If she'd stopped long enough to hear my reply, she would have heard me say: 'No, I haven't stopped.' But then she wasn't particularly interested in what I had to say.

It made me feel rotten. Two months after returning to work, when Betty was fourteen months, I told Will I didn't think I could carry on expressing.

'It's hard enough to get our breaks these days, let alone

Changes

arrange cover for twenty minutes while I express,' I told him. 'They just make me feel so bad about doing it.'

'It's fine,' he soothed. 'You've done an amazing job. You've gone above and beyond with the feeding, Pip, and let's face it, it hasn't been easy for you with the mastitis. So just don't worry about it.'

'I know. I just wish I had stopped of my own accord.'

All in all, I really didn't have much to complain about. I was pleased to be back at work, among my friends and colleagues, doing the job I loved. Of course there were changes, but nothing I couldn't handle. And, as before, no two days were the same.

* * *

One crisp September morning, the police brought in an Indian lady in the late stages of pregnancy. She seemed well-mannered and polite, but incredibly frightened, her eyes darting to the door whenever she heard it bang open. The police explained that they had brought Parvan from Birmingham, as she was on Witness Protection. Parvan was originally from India, but the previous year she had married into an Indian family based in the UK in a formally arranged marriage ceremony. She had never even set eyes on her husband before she flew out to live with him and his relatives in Birmingham. And no sooner had she arrived than her dreams of a happily married life crumbled before her eyes. Her husband was a brute, and his family were cruel and violent. From the word go, they had kept Parvan prisoner in their home. She was never allowed outside the home; they had starved her and prevented her from having any contact with friends and family. It was only when she developed gestational diabetes that they were forced to take her to the GP surgery, and that's when a terrified Parvan revealed to the midwives that she was being held captive.

She was interviewed by police, and the family were subsequently arrested and charged with false imprisonment. Incredibly, as soon as the husband was released on police bail, he went straight to the hospital and made threats on Parvan's life. It had happened right in front of the hospital staff, so now the police couldn't take any chances. Parvan was immediately moved out of the area and placed in a secure house in our city. Then, a few hours after she arrived at the secure house, she alerted the emergency services, convinced her waters had gone, and was brought onto our ward.

When we looked her over, however, we found her waters were still intact, which was just as well, as she was still only thirty-seven weeks. However, we decided that, because of the diabetes, it would be safest to keep her on the ward until her due date. This appeared to suit Parvan, who was very frightened and relieved not to be sent back to the safe house. I think she craved the comfort and security of being around other people. Still, she was so nervous she was afraid to sleep with the lights off. The police had given her a new identity and we were under strict instructions not to let anyone onto the ward who could be connected with the family. We had to contact the police immediately if anyone came in and gave Parvan's old name. Even the police officers that came to the ward needed to give us a special code word to allow them access to her.

At first, Parvan was so timid she wouldn't talk to us at all. We didn't even know if she spoke English because she was too frightened to open her mouth. But gradually, over time, she learned to trust us and, during the quiet nights on the ward, she opened up. Parvan said she had come from a good family in India and had worked as an accountant before marrying and moving to the UK. It was meant to be a wonderful opportunity to start a new life, but her husband's family had treated her badly from the start. They locked her in her room, feeding her one meal a day at most, while at night her new husband regularly raped her. She was kept a prisoner in the home, without access to a phone or computer.

'Every now and then, they let me come downstairs,' she said in her soft Indian accent. 'But when I did, they said I had to sit on the small bench and not move or talk. And if I didn't obey their rules, the family would beat me.'

'Who? Who beat you?' I asked.

'All of them,' she said simply. 'My husband, the mother, father, and even my brother-in-law. They didn't let me call my family in India, and when I got pregnant they told me that if the baby was a girl, they would kill us both, and if it was a boy, they would take the child and kill me. I was terrified. I didn't know what to do.'

'Were there any visitors to the house?'

'Sometimes at the weekend the family visited, but if I was allowed out then I had to just sit on the bench and not even look them in the eyes. What could I do? If I said anything to the family they would just beat me. I wanted to escape but I didn't know where I was, or how to get help. I didn't know the name of the streets or how to get anywhere. Especially being pregnant . . . I couldn't just run away and sleep on the streets. It wasn't until they took me to see the doctor that I found a way to get help.'

The Secret Midwife

Parvan was worried that her husband was now out on bail, but the police assured her that he had no information on her whereabouts – still, no amount of reassurance would calm her fears.

'We have security cameras,' I told her, pointing up at the little black boxes in the corners of the room. 'All the doors are locked, and there's always a receptionist here.'

'I know, I know . . . but you don't know these people.'

'Would they really kill you?'

'Of course,' she replied without hesitation. 'It's a matter of honour. If I give evidence in court against them, their family honour will be destroyed.'

Over the next three weeks, we all got close to Parvan. She was a lovely lady – so kind and gentle – and we felt very sorry that she didn't know a soul in this town. It was bizarre, but at that moment we midwives were the closest thing she had to a family.

A week before the birth, we threw her a baby shower, chipping in to get her everything she would need for her new child. After all, she had come to us with nothing but the clothes she stood up in. So, after a whip-round, we bought her sleepsuits, nappies, bottles, vests and other bits and bobs – all wrapped up in a huge baby hamper. When we gave it to her, she was so moved she could barely speak.

'I am overwhelmed by this kindness,' she said, smiling through her tears. 'After suffering such cruelty, it means so much. You give me faith again that there are good people in this world. You are all good people. Thank you.'

In the safe world of our labour ward, Parvan had blossomed and become a friend to us all. Occasionally, she borrowed a laptop from one of the coordinators and Skyped

Changes

her family back in India, telling them all about us and how well she was being cared for. When her little girl was born by C-section, we were all there for her and, eventually, she was allowed to take her baby back to the safe house. It was such a sad day when she left us. She took lots of photos – 'So that one day I can show my daughter the people who cared for us in our hour of need.'

Parvan's brother was due to fly from India to help with the baby, and I really hoped that he would look after them both. Parvan left us with a smile and words of optimism – she said that despite what she went through she loved being in the UK and was looking forward to building a new life for herself and her daughter here. We didn't hear from her again after that, but I still think about her a lot. I think about how brave she had been in facing up to her abusive husband and his family, and how much hope she had for the future.

* * *

As midwives, we are fully aware of the issues surrounding domestic abuse, and we get safeguarding updates every year. We are trained to look out for the signs of domestic abuse and controlling, coercive behaviour – like a man always speaking for his partner, or a woman's fearful looks or careful reaction around their husband or boyfriend. Then, if we have suspicions, we'll try to arrange a moment with the woman on her own, to ask if they have anything to disclose. Sometimes they tell you, sometimes they don't. But even if they admit their partner is violent, whether they want to do anything about it is another matter. It can be very frustrating but we do what we can. You can only give

173

them the advice that's there, hand them the relevant contact details and leave it up to them to follow through.

A year after returning to work after having Betty, I was back into the swing of things. And though motherhood hadn't changed me as a midwife, I felt much more sympathetic to the women in pain, keen to offer them as much relief as they needed. I was also eager to help with breastfeeding support, given how difficult it had been for me to feed once Betty had fallen sick. Between us, Will and I juggled the childcare: I did three twelve-hour shifts a week in order to look after her at the weekend; Will managed his hours to take off a day a week for Betty, while my mum also helped out. Then, from eighteen months, Betty went to nursery for one long day and one half-day a week, with my parents sharing the pick-ups and drops-offs.

As much as I wanted to, I couldn't stay the extra hours at work any more. The demands of parenthood meant I could no longer do tons of overtime after my shift ended the way I used to. Of course, I still wanted to give my all to every birthing mother that came onto the ward, but Betty needed me too. And having my own family meant prioritising their needs. Still, there are some experiences you share with a family that bond you together in a way that goes far beyond a 'professional' relationship. And though you cherish your precious days off, there are times when you willingly give these up because you know it is the right thing to do. Sadly, most often, these are for funerals.

14

Small Mercies

I'd spotted the sunny daffodils on my way into work that morning and couldn't resist – they looked so bright and cheerful. It was early March, and for the previous two days I'd been looking after a lovely same-sex couple in their thirties – Jade and Marion. Jade had had a sperm donor insemination and was pregnant at thirty-seven weeks with their little girl when a routine scan revealed the devastating news that their baby had died. Unable to cope with the idea of a vaginal birth, Jade had opted for a C-section, and myself and my student midwife Katie had been the ones to look after them during this tragic event. They were two of the loveliest people I'd ever met, and though the past forty-eight hours had been probably the worst of their lives, they had handled the experience with honesty, grace and a shedload of humour. Now, after handover, I went to our bereavement suite, where Jade and Marion were staying.

'Morning,' I said, after knocking and gently opening the door. 'Brought you something.'

The Secret Midwife

I held out the bunch of yellow flowers.

'Oh, are those for us?' Jade grinned at me from the bed.

'Yes, just something to brighten this place up a bit.'

'How lovely! Thank you. I'm sure we can rustle up a mug to put them in.'

'I'm on it.' Marion busied herself, retrieving a mug from the kitchen and filling it with water.

'How are we doing this morning?' I asked.

'Not bad.' Jade smiled, rubbing her shaved head. 'Up and down.'

It had been like that with these two the whole time – one minute they'd be crying their eyes out and the next they were laughing their heads off at something silly. The emotions in that room were raw and wild, but they were always loving and in tune with one another. I had to admire their courage in being so honest with their feelings. Not all couples coped so well. When their little girl – Annie – was born, Jade and Marion were overcome with love and couldn't stop cuddling her. The place was awash with tears, but there were also moments of genuine happiness. Both mums thought Annie's feet looked huge.

'She has got flippers for feet,' Marion insisted.

'Our little princess,' Jade said, grinning. 'Look at the size of them! Takes after you!'

There was no knot in the cord, and all of Annie's blood tests came back normal, so we had no clear idea of why she had died in utero, but both Jade and Marion were adamant they didn't want a post-mortem. To them, Annie was perfect, and they didn't want her 'messed around with'. Her death was simply an unexplained tragedy and they were content to leave it at that. She stayed in the cool cot in the suite with them and they cherished the short time they could share with her, inviting all members of the family to come in and have a cuddle.

'Erm, Pippa, we've got to ask you something,' Jade now started. Marion came back and sat down on the bed next to Jade and the pair instinctively linked hands.

'We'd like to invite you to the funeral,' Marion said. 'It's a week on Tuesday. We do understand that this isn't strictly . . .'

'Oh yes, of course I'll come,' I said quickly. 'I'd love to. I'll go and have a look at the rota now and make sure I can get the time off.' I dashed off immediately to check. There was no doubt in my mind that I would go to Annie's funeral. After all, I was one of the few people who had spent time with her, and I knew how much it meant to Jade and Marion for me to be there.

In my many years as a midwife, I had already attended dozens of baby funerals, though it isn't something they tell you about in training. And why would they? Officially, this isn't part of the job. So when I was invited to my first baby funeral within a few months of qualifying, I wasn't sure at first if I should go. *Was it the right thing to do? Did it cross the line between 'professional' and overly familiar?* I worried about what to do. Doctors don't go to baby funerals. They don't go to funerals full stop. If a doctor had just pronounced a ninety-year-old woman dead, he wouldn't consider going to her funeral. But with midwifery it's different. You might be one of the only people who has held that baby or seen them alive. You might have formed a strong bond with the family. It didn't take long for me to make up my mind – I knew I wanted to show my respects to the family and to bear witness to that child's life and death. I went to that first funeral and have been to every single one since for which I've received an invite.

These days, I attend around four or five baby funerals a year, but it never fails to move me when I see the tiny coffin being brought in, sometimes no bigger than a shoebox, often decorated with daisies, butterflies or teddies drawn on by older siblings. I imagine these will be small, intimate ceremonies, but many times I've been surprised by a packed crematorium with standing room only. So much love for a life that nobody has known. Together we mourn the child that could have been. I always wonder what happens afterwards. How does the family cope? They've spent so much time getting ready for their baby: buying clothes, equipment, buggies, planning their room, picking a name – and then, there's nothing. I always imagine that is the hardest time. The first time they go home after the funeral, and walk into the baby's room, look inside and see the empty cot.

Katie and I went to Annie's funeral together. As a student, this had been her first stillborn experience and it had affected her very deeply. Until that point she had been recording the number of boys and girls she had helped deliver by putting pink and blue buttons in a jar. But for Annie, she sewed tiny wings onto a pink button and threaded her name onto a little loop underneath. When Katie brought this in to show Jade and Marion, they were moved to tears. The four of us, in fact, had become very close over the three days they stayed in our bereavement suite, and Katie and I went out of our way to give them the best experience they could have considering the circumstances. If we went for a coffee, we'd bring two back for Jade and Marion; we brought them flowers, small gifts and we helped them make footprint casts of Annie's feet, so they had a permanent reminder of her large flipper feet! Small gestures, but meaningful. There's nothing you can do to change the terrible fact that they have lost their child, but we try our best to make the pain of their loss as bearable as possible.

Theirs was a beautiful ceremony. There were poems, songs and readings, and Marion had even written a fairy story about their princess, the daughter of the royal queens, who had been 'born asleep'. Katie and I even featured in the story as the royal matrons. It ended with the emotional line '. . . even though the princess had been born asleep, the gentle smile on her lips told the queens that her dreams were happy ones'. It was tender, sweet and utterly heartbreaking, and when Marion read the story aloud, we were all in floods of tears. Marion and Jade had asked all the funeral guests to bring a soft toy to hold during the ceremony, and now I gripped Betty's giraffe tightly to my chest as I took in long, shaky breaths. The crematorium was packed to bursting, and I was astonished to see there were six members of staff from the hospital in total – four midwives, a healthcare assistant and Sheila, the ODP. Some families are just like that; they leave their mark on many hearts. As I looked around me, taking in the family and friends along with my colleagues, it reminded me once again how the role of a midwife does not exist solely within the walls of a hospital, but within the community with the families who we meet along the way.

Of course I was thrilled when, a year later, Jade and Marion dropped by to share the good news – a twelve-week baby scan! They had been frequent visitors to the hospital since Annie's birth, as members of our bereavement group, but during that time they had also been trying for another child through sperm donation, and now Marion had fallen pregnant. Thankfully, the pregnancy went smoothly, though towards the end they were in and out of the ward with various worries. Unsurprisingly, it was an anxious time and they both needed a lot of reassurance. Fearful of history repeating itself, Marion was induced just after thirty-seven weeks, and their beautiful little girl Alice was born. It was so wonderful to see this gorgeous family blessed with another little girl and, from the word go, Annie was a presence in Alice's life. Jade and Marion had put her ashes inside a cuddly toy and given it to Alice so that they could always be 'together'. In this way, Alice's birth had also become an act of remembrance for Annie.

'She was our daughter, just as much as Alice,' Jade insisted. 'We're never going to forget her. She'll always be a part of our family.'

Today, all the midwives on our ward who know Jade and Marion maintain a strong relationship with them both. I suppose we are an important part of their family history because we were among the few people who met Annie. We were part of 'Annie's world' and our chaplain became so attached to Jade and Marion that he bought Alice a silver bracelet as a christening gift.

As a society, we tend to forget about stillborn babies, the ones that never made it, but they are always present in their mothers' and fathers' hearts. They never forget, even if to the outside world they don't appear to exist. I've delivered hundreds of healthy babies in the town where I live, and I always say 'Hi' to those mums if I see them in the street. But if I see a mum whose baby didn't make it, I make a point of stopping to chat to her, too. I remember their child even if nobody else does. I remember what happened in that room, in that moment between life and death, hope and despair, joy and pain. It's not much to ask – just to acknowledge their child's life – and for most people, the fact that you are willing to share their grief means a great deal. However, not everybody reacts in the same way to the loss of a child. For some, the pain is too much to bear and what they can't accept turns into anger.

* * *

Not long after Jade and Marion had Alice, I was put in charge of a woman called Sally who, at eighteen years old, was pregnant with her first baby. Sally was thirty-nine weeks and had come in one Sunday morning in the very early stages of labour, complaining that she couldn't cope with the pain at home. She was still only 2 cms, so we gave her some diamorphine to keep the worst of the pain at bay and put her and her boyfriend Rylie in a room to rest. That lasted around four hours, but soon Sally was crying out for pain relief once more, begging for an epidural. Since she wasn't yet in what we call established labour (that means over 4 cms dilated) we couldn't give her an epidural. This was a tricky one. I called in the registrar for a consultation.

'The contractions are still fairly irregular,' I explained, 'but they're obviously stronger than she can cope with. We've had her in the pool, we've given her some food, tried her with the aromatherapy oils, but she's still saying she is in a great deal of pain. What do you think?'

'It's a long latent phase, isn't it?' the registrar said, looking over Sally's notes. 'I suggest we break her waters to try and move things along, and in the meantime, we give her some more pain relief.'

I organised another diamorphine injection and, at 7 p.m., I went through handover with the night-time staff, giving them the doctor's instruction to break Sally's waters.

When I started my next shift at 7 p.m. the following evening, I was shocked and upset to be told during handover that Sally's baby had been a fresh stillborn. I listened intently as the LWC explained that Sally's waters were broken in the early hours – at that point there was no signs anything was amiss. The monitor showed the baby's heartbeat was fine, and Sally was started on the hormone drip and given an epidural. By late afternoon Sally was fully dilated and pushing, but to no effect. Still, all the signs were normal, and she was taken into theatre for a forceps delivery, but on delivery there was no heartbeat on the little boy, and he failed to take a single breath. Full resuscitation was carried out, the baby was intubated, but he was pronounced dead at 6.30 p.m. At this stage the medical team had no idea why the baby died.

'Pippa, you know this lady,' Jen said. 'I think it best if you look after her.' I nodded solemnly. Poor Sally – she had laboured for so long. I made sure I went to see her straight after handover.

She was holding her little boy when I came into the room. She looked pale, stricken and suddenly very, very young.

'I'm so sorry, Sally,' I said.

'It's alright,' she said mechanically. She was still in shock – after all, the birth had taken place just an hour before. Until that moment, everything had been fine. The father, Rylie, now shouldered his way past me to the door and muttered, 'Going out for a fag,' as he left.

'He's beautiful,' I said, sitting down on the bed next to her and looking closely at the still, lifeless child in her arms. There was a heavy silence in the room. Then . . .

'I . . . I just . . . I can't believe it,' she stammered. 'How do I tell people? How do I tell my family? Will you ring them for me? Please?' This took me by surprise. Nobody had ever asked me to do this for them.

'I *can* do, Sally,' I started reluctantly. 'But don't you think it's best coming from you?'

'I can't. I just can't. I want them to meet him but I can't be the one that rings them.' Suddenly it hit me that Sally was still just a youngster herself – a teenager – she didn't know how to handle the situation.

I agreed to make the call to Sally's mother, who picked up straight away, clearly waiting for good news.

'My name is Pippa,' I said slowly, my heart thumping in my chest. 'I'm a midwife at the hospital looking after your daughter, and she's asked me to call you because, sadly, the baby has passed away – but Sally wants you to come into hospital. She wants you to meet the baby.'

There was a sharp intake of breath, followed by, 'What do you mean? What do you *mean*?'

'Like I said, the baby has passed away.'

'What are you *talking about*? What the *fuck* are you talking about? DEAD? HOW CAN HE BE DEAD? HOW?'

Sally's mother was livid. I didn't quite know how to reply, so I said, 'Your daughter is asking you to come in to be there for her. That's all I can say right now.' When I hung up, my heart was pounding and I felt a knot of dread forming in the pit of my stomach.

The family arrived on the ward half an hour later and they were furious, absolutely furious. I was desperate to calm them down, for Sally's sake, but it seemed no matter what I said it only riled them up further. There were eight of them – the mother, grandmother, father and several aunts and uncles – all firing questions at me at once.

'What happened?'

'Why did she have forceps?'

'Why was she allowed to go so long?'

'Why didn't someone do something earlier?'

'I can only tell you what I've been told,' I said, trying to sound emollient. 'I wasn't actually there at the birth.'

'Well, who was there?' the mother demanded to know. 'Who can give us some bloody answers?'

'I'll go and get a doctor to come and talk to you,' I said, and rushed off to find the registrar who had conducted the delivery in theatre. But when I got to the staffroom, I found Dr Hadip on the sofa being comforted by an ODP. He was in pieces.

'Can you come and talk to this family, please? They are asking for further information.'

'I don't know. I just don't know what happened. I don't know . . . did I make the right decision? I can't. I just can't.' He shook his head and looked away.

'The family need briefing,' I insisted. 'Someone needs to talk to them.'

'The night-time registrar,' he mumbled. 'I'll update her and she can talk to them.'

So, after Dr Hadip updated the night-time registrar, she

went down to the ward and explained as much as she knew to the family. I felt sorry for Sally – she needed rest and comfort, but her family were getting her all worked up. They still weren't placated and kept on at me for answers. In search of further support, I enlisted the help of the paediatrician who had been in theatre to explain what he knew about the birth. Unfortunately, the message was the same from all of us: at this stage we had no idea why the baby had died, and the next step was to investigate exactly what happened.

'We can do blood tests,' I explained. 'We'll send the placenta away for tests; we'll do a post-mortem. We'll take all necessary steps to get the answers you deserve. I understand you're upset and angry but really, there's nothing more I can say at this point.'

They all looked at me in disgust, standing around the bed in the middle of the room, surrounding their daughter, niece and grandchild, as if for protection, but in a way that seemed very intimidating. Each one of them looked to me for answers, and they weren't happy that I didn't have any. Nevertheless, the questions kept coming. No matter what I said, it just wasn't enough. Yes, I was the official face of the hospital, but I couldn't help any further and, as I kept explaining, I wasn't actually present during the birth itself. Jen finally explained to them that I couldn't answer any more questions, and, in the early hours, we managed to persuade them to leave in order to give Sally some rest. I was completely drained afterwards.

Of course, the family submitted a formal complaint immediately, and I was astonished when I read that Sally had taken my words 'I'm so sorry' – which I had said when

I first entered her room – as an *apology* for something we'd done wrong. Whereas, I just meant 'sorry' in the sense of expressing *regret* for what she had suffered on a human level. At the same time, the hospital conducted its own review, anticipating that the coroner would need further information to determine the cause of death. The hospital solicitors questioned me, as the family had claimed Sally had been given nothing to eat all day on Sunday. Fortunately, it was documented in my notes that Sally ate a couple of pieces of toast. But the investigations took time, of course, and meanwhile I went about my life.

About two months after Sally's baby died, I was out with Betty and my mum. We'd just been to Asda to buy a few bits for our tea and were walking back to Mum's house with Betty in the pushchair. But as we stopped by the traffic lights, I noticed Sally's family standing on the other side of the road. They were looking at me with venom, muttering and pointing in my direction. Suddenly, Rylie shouted out: 'YOU'RE A MURDERER!'

I turned to Mum and, as quietly as I could, whispered, 'Mum, Mum, they're talking about me! That's the woman who lost her baby.'

Now Rylie was shouting at me from the other side of the street: 'YOU KILLED MY BABY!' And a couple of the others were also shouting, 'MURDERER!'

'What do we do?' I started to panic. They were there on the street, away from the security of the hospital ward. I felt very vulnerable. *What would they do to me if they got to my side of the road? Would they attack me? What about Betty?*

'Come on!' Mum took me by the arm and quickly steered us away from the lights. We walked swiftly in the other direction, taking the long route home, but I was constantly looking round, checking they weren't following us. My heart was going at a million miles an hour, blood roaring through my ears. I felt like I was going to faint. I wanted to run but I couldn't with Betty in the pushchair. *What if they follow us home? What do we do?* My whole body was shaking as we arrived at my mum's house and, once we had the door shut firmly behind us, I fell into her arms, weeping.

'I've never been so scared in my life,' I said. 'I thought they were going to attack us. What should I do?'

'You should tell your managers about this. They can't behave like this! Shouting at you in the street, scaring you. It's not on.'

So promptly, as soon as I came on shift the next day, I requested a private meeting with one of the Navy Blues. It was Lina, the one who had told me off about the socks.

'They called me a murderer, in front of my mum and daughter,' I said. 'I thought they were going to physically attack me. It was awful. I'm worried they know where we live and I'm scared even to leave the house.'

She nodded brusquely. 'Well, it's all over now. Next time something like that happens, call the police.'

'Well, yes, but . . .'

'That's really what you ought to do.'

'Oh, okay.'

'Was there anything else?'

'Erm, no.'

And that was it – I walked out of her office feeling just as terrible as when I walked in. Probably worse, because now I knew I had no support from the management. I was constantly on alert over the next few weeks, checking the street before I left the house, careful not to go out in public spaces and remaining vigilant all night long, terrified the family were going to put my windows through. Fortunately, nothing happened, and I eventually stopped living my life in fear.

* * *

The coroner's inquest for Sally's baby was heard a year after his death and, unfortunately for her, the investigations proved inconclusive. Despite the family's insistence on medical negligence, the coroner found there was no clear evidence as to what caused the baby to die and recorded an open verdict. A couple of midwives who had been present during the birth were called to give evidence in court, but were ushered out early as there were concerns for their safety because of threats made by the family. Apparently, the family's solicitor had demanded to know why I hadn't given evidence in court, but as was explained to them, I hadn't actually been present at the birth, so my evidence was not useful. I was relieved not to have to go to court or to face that family again; it shook me up so much. But I felt for Sally – she never got to find out why her baby hadn't lived.

A couple of years later, Sally fell pregnant again and had a healthy baby girl, born in a different hospital. Another happy ending. Although I'm sure she was thrilled to have a live child, I knew that nothing could possibly take away the pain of that first loss. I never forgot her or her family, and whenever I saw an entry on our bookings system of the same surname, I was petrified it was them. People react in many different ways to pain of losing a child. I do understand that anger is a natural part of the grieving process, and I wish they had got the answers they sought. But there was no excuse for the vicious abuse and nasty threats directed at myself and the other midwives. To frighten me on the street in that way, while I had my baby daughter with me, was unjustifiable. It was the first time I had encountered real anger directed at me – but the thing that lingered most in my mind was just how little support the hospital had offered. When I needed them most, *where were they*?

15

Sam

S am was off sick with stress and I was sad for her, but angry at the same time. *It's not right what they've done to her. It's just not right.* I walked into the staffroom and there, on the whiteboard, was a patronising handwritten note to staff: 'Please remember you are not qualified to use the ultrasound scanner unless you have received additional training' – with a laminated copy of the guidelines hanging below.

'Bastards!' I exclaimed and, in a fit of anger, I wiped the board clean.

'Careful there,' Angela warned. 'You don't want them to catch you messing up all their nice work.'

'I don't care,' I fumed. 'That's a horrible thing to do. We all know who this is aimed at, and it's not right to put it up on the wall to humiliate her in front of everyone. Don't you think she's been through enough?'

'I agree with you, darling,' Angela said, and shook her head. 'Sam doesn't deserve that sort of treatment.'

The Secret Midwife

'No. She's a bloody good midwife and all of this is totally unfair.'

It had started three weeks ago when Sam had been assigned to look after a woman, Clare, who was twenty-six weeks pregnant. Clare was what we would class as 'pre-term', but her waters had broken and it looked like she was in labour. Of course, with any pre-termer the risks during delivery are higher than if the pregnancy had gone to full term – a fully mature baby copes better with the stress of delivery, and their lungs are better equipped to breathe on their own – so Sam requested help from the doctors. Unfortunately, the registrar was in the middle of a forceps delivery and the consultant was in main theatre, so neither could attend.

Clare had been quite happy at first, but as the labour progressed, she felt she couldn't cope and wanted more pain relief. Things were getting to a crucial stage but there was still no sign of either doctor. Sam knew the first thing the doctor would want to see was an ultrasound scan, to discover the presentation of the baby, but there was nobody around qualified to do a scan. Sam was in a state of panic – what to do? She knew the woman was going to be delivering soon, and she needed to know where the baby was. So she wheeled in the ultrasound scanner herself and carried out a scan, discovering that the baby was breech, which meant the birth was even more risky, as the baby would come out bottom first. By this time, Clare was bearing down and she wanted to push. As a last-ditch effort, Sam made another round of requests for a doctor to attend, but with the two on our ward still taken up with other women, she was left to manage this risky birth alone.

192

Sam

The baby came out bottom first just as the registrar came into the room, but then, before it was fully delivered, the cervix clamped round the baby's neck. With pre-termers, the baby is so small it can slip through the cervix even when it's not fully dilated. In this case it had obviously stretched just enough for the body but shrunk back down again before the head came out. The doctor and Sam tried everything to get this baby delivered but he just wasn't coming. In the end the doctor attempted to cut the cervix, but by the time the baby delivered it had died. Naturally the family were distraught, but from the word go, the finger of blame was pointed very firmly in Sam's direction. The Navy Blues told the family that Sam was not qualified to use the scanner and, if she had not done so, they would have a live baby.

Sam was hauled into Lina's office and told to pack her bags because she was going to lose her job due to the decisions she had made. Sam was so distraught she had to leave the ward in the middle of her shift. Of course, there would be an investigation, and Sam was in theory innocent until proven guilty, but from the way the Navy Blues behaved it was an open and shut case – Sam had been hung out to dry.

We were close friends, Sam and I, and had actually become closer in the last couple of years, as our children were the same age and we'd started going on playdates together. We spoke many times about her situation. I was horrified at the way she was being treated. Now the family had somehow got hold of her Facebook details and were sending her nasty messages.

'I just don't understand it,' I said one night when we were on shift together. 'Even though you weren't meant to use the scanner, it made absolutely no difference to the outcome of the birth. The only thing that would have made a difference would have been if you'd managed to get a doctor to review her earlier.'

'I know!' she said. 'This baby was coming and I had no one else to do it. The ward was very short-staffed and the LWC was busy assisting with the other two emergencies on the ward at the same time. What exactly am I meant to do when I'm in that situation and there's nobody more senior to help? Either way, though, the baby didn't die because of the scan.'

Things only worsened for Sam over the next couple of weeks. Clare's family had joined our hospital bereavement group, and Sam was told they were hounding another family to get hold of Sam's home address.

She explained: 'I gave my address to a lovely bereaved family when I printed out some pictures for them on my home printer. The hospital printer was broken at the time.' I nodded and rolled my eyes. Broken printers were the bane of our existence.

'Well, anyway, somehow Clare got wind of the fact that the nice family had my home address, and now she keeps asking them for it. They told me, as they thought I should know.'

'Have you told the Navy Blues?'

'Of course. They said there was nothing they could do.'

'Oh, for heaven's sake!'

'It's just now I don't feel safe in my home any more. I keep worrying they're going to turn up one day. And what with the baby . . .' Sam put a protective hand over her bump. 'It's just all getting too much.'

Sam

I knew exactly what she meant. I had been through the same thing with Sally's family only six months earlier. And look how much protection the hospital had given me then! But Sam was getting more and more freaked out and it wasn't good for her own pregnancy. Eventually, she called me up one evening to say I wouldn't be seeing her on the ward as she was now signed off work with stress.

I didn't hear from Sam again for another five months. Phone calls went unanswered and texts disappeared without replies, but of course we talked about her at work during this time. When her baby girl was born, we sent flowers and a card but still we heard nothing. It was upsetting – we were a close-knit group and we were always there for one another during the hard times. With Sam gone it was like losing a member of our little family, and we worried and fretted about how she was coping. One day, in the staffroom, I wondered aloud whether she would ever come back to the ward.

'I suppose it depends what happens with the case,' Bev replied.

'That's enough gossiping from you lot!' one of the Navy Blues admonished.

'It's not gossiping,' I countered. 'She's our friend and we're worried about her.'

'Well, that sounds like gossip and that won't help your friend one bit.'

'Rubbish! If we talk about these things openly, maybe we can improve our practices and procedures.'

I was so cross. They wanted to hush it all up, to sweep it under the carpet. But the management – who should have been behind Sam from the start – were in the process of ruining the unblemished career of a brilliant midwife. And, funnily enough, I didn't feel like staying quiet about it all.

Finally, eight months after she went off with stress, I got a text message from Sam that made me smile: 'Fancy a playdate in the park? Want to meet Ruby?'

I couldn't get Betty in her stroller quickly enough, and when I arrived at the cafe next to the play park, I was relieved to see Sam looking healthier and happier than I'd seen in ages. In the pram next to her was a gorgeous four-month-old girl – Ruby!

'Can I?' I asked excitedly.

'Of course!' She smiled and I dug my hands in and lifted out the gorgeous little bundle. She had that lovely warm biscuity smell of breast-fed babies, and was bonny and attractively plump. I enjoyed the weightiness of her in my arms, and Sam looked on, clearly besotted with her little girl. Now Sam's eldest boy Barney, and Betty – who were both three – made a beeline for the climbing frame while we grabbed a coffee and sat outside, watching our kids play together.

'So, how've you been?' I started.

'Better now, thanks. I'm so sorry I haven't been in touch, but it's actually been a really tough time. Did you hear about the investigation?'

'Yes! No evidence of negligence. You were cleared.'

'I was cleared,' she repeated with a hollow laugh. 'After all that, I was cleared! The Trust found that even though I had used the scanner, which I wasn't qualified to do, it had no impact on the outcome of the birth.'

'Which we already knew!'

'Well, *we* knew it, but the family didn't. Before I went off sick, they were bombarding me with Facebook messages every day. I tried to block them but they were emailing me too, so I had to change my email address. Meanwhile, I was a complete mess! I was terrified of losing my job. I put on a brave face as much I could, but I was worried *all the time*. I felt like I was being watched, that the management were breathing down my neck, just waiting for me to make another slip up, giving them an excuse to suspend me, willing me to write my resignation. I felt like they were talking about me constantly and I got very paranoid at work. That's when the doctor signed me off with stress. So then I was sat at home, heavily-pregnant, petrified all the time, worried about the family tracking me down, worried about losing my job, and I stopped sleeping. I wasn't eating properly. I cried all the time. I just got more and more stressed, and that's when I started to hallucinate. Then I was admitted to the psychiatric unit.'

'What? No!'

'It was probably the best place for me at the time. It gave me a bit of respite because I was getting so worried at home. They put me on antidepressants and I got some counselling, and that all helped too. I was in there for a couple of weeks before I came home, and by then I had contacted the union. They were great. They told me that Lina's behaviour was completely unacceptable. I should never have been told I was going to lose my job, and the family should never have been told the baby died because of me. They took up my case and that made things a lot easier. You know, with Dan only pulling in a gardener's wage, losing my job would have destroyed us financially. I don't think we could have coped.'

'Oh God, Sam, I'm so sorry.'

'Thanks. Yeah, it's been tough.'

Together we watched silently as our children rocked back and forth on the seesaw. I was trying to get my head round it all. I couldn't believe my friend had been driven to a breakdown by all of this. And now she was on antidepressants? It didn't make any sense.

'I'm coming back, you know,' she said, grinning at me. 'Yeah, I can't believe I'm such a glutton for punishment either, but, to be honest, I need to work. At least I have a job to go back to.'

* * *

Sam returned to the ward two months later, but it was clear from the outset that the trauma had left its mark on her. She was cautious, timid, constantly calling in the doctors for minor concerns that she would have been able to handle on her own before the scanner incident. Sam used to be the confident one among us – now she was constantly asking us all what we would do. It made me sad to see how much she had changed. She confided to me that she had upped her antidepressant dosage and had a stash of anti-anxiety pills to take whenever she felt it all getting on top of her. The investigation now resolved there was no further action to be taken against the hospital or any individual practitioners. And yet, I couldn't forget how Sam had been treated. She deserved compensation for everything they put her through – an apology at the least. But no, nothing. For all the pain and misery Lina had caused, she was never reprimanded and never once offered anything approaching an apology. It was extraordinary to me that she could derail Sam's life so thoroughly and suffer no consequences as a result. I couldn't help it – I was really beginning to resent our hospital management.

Don't get me wrong: I still loved being a midwife and our team was fantastic. It wasn't always easy but we got through it together – we laughed, we cried, we ate pizza – and whenever anyone needed a hand, we were all there for each other. Not just midwives – doctors, health care support workers, breastfeeding support workers, receptionists, anaesthetists too. We were a team, and when it worked, it worked so well. But it was clear there was a growing feeling of alienation between midwives and those who managed us. The main problem seemed to be their physical distance from the ward. They hardly ever came onto the unit, so we had no relationship with any of them. If they did come onto the ward, they wouldn't communicate with us, only the Labour Ward Coordinators. Everything was now done through email. If there were new guidelines, or a change in policy, you'd be sent an email with an attachment. There was precious little opportunity to give any feedback from our side of things, but they didn't hesitate to relay criticism from patients.

Every decision seemed to be about money. For the very first time in my professional life, we actually had to close the ward to new admissions. It was only a six-hour closure but it was a shock to be told that we could no longer take any further admissions for 'patient safety'.

'If we only had some more bloody midwives and a few less managers we'd be fine,' I remarked to Helen one day. It was so frustrating to close the ward – for one thing, it meant a midwife had to sit on the phone in order to redirect the calls to other hospitals. That alone took up a practitioner.

'You know, we're three midwives down today,' Helen said, munching on her chicken salad sandwich.

'Of course we are – everyone's off with sickness and stress from being constantly understaffed and overworked. I've been on for eight hours already and this is my first break.'

At that very moment, a Navy Blue wandered in. I was shocked – you never usually saw them on the ward. Was she lost? She'd clearly heard this last moan of mine because she shot me a look. A warm blush spread from my neck right up to my ears. I was embarrassed, but at the same time I thought: *Good! They never usually hear this sort of thing. They never ask us what we think. Maybe it's about time they heard the truth.*

The truth was we were coming under increasing strain to do more and more for less and less. By now we were all under a public sector pay freeze, thanks to the financial crisis, so our wage packets had to stretch further while inflation kept rising. And whenever there was a problem, it seemed that us midwives were always the first to get the blame. I had never heard of a doctor being reprimanded for failure to attend (I still haven't!) and yet we can be given a rap on the knuckles for failing to ask enough times for the doctor to come. It was ridiculous. I once telephoned the 'on call' consultant because we had a case of bradycardia – when a baby's heartbeat slows right down and takes time to get back up again. In these situations, it's a very finely balanced decision whether to give the woman a C-section or try to deliver the baby vaginally. The registrar was unsure of how to proceed and needed advice from a more senior member of the team, so I rang up the consultant.

'Sorry, I can't come,' he replied. 'I'm at a black-tie do. But don't worry, I've covered it. Let me give you my colleague's number. She's going to cover for me tonight.'

He was ON CALL, for heaven's sake. That meant wherever he was – a black-tie do, a funfair or his own bloody wedding – he should have come without question. It took two more hours to get hold of his nominated stand-in, by which time we managed to get the baby out safe and sound, but it was touch and go for a time, and I dreaded to think what would have happened if we had encountered a serious problem. In that case, I believe the consultant was in breach of his duty of care. He should have left the black-tie ball and come to the hospital. That's what being 'on call' means.

Generally speaking, we don't see the consultants all that much. They come in during the morning for the ward round, then they vanish, and everything is left to the registrar or the SHO. But they do have their bleepers, so we can ring them if we need them. At night, some may come in for the night-time review, but most don't. I have to say that, mostly, we have very good relationships with the consultants, and they are there for advice if we need them, but if something does go wrong, they are very quick to pass the blame.

One time, I was attending a forceps delivery and the baby was quite high in the pelvis. The strict rule with forceps is 'three pulls MAXIMUM', but I watched the registrar take FIVE pulls to try to get this baby out.

After the third pull, Jen asked, 'Do you think we need to go for a C-section?'

'No, it's coming, this baby's coming,' the registrar insisted. And then he tried again. These doctors have years of experience and are extremely intelligent, so you don't question their methods more than once, but this was terrible. Jen and I looked at one another, alarmed.

'Are we doing a C-section?' she asked again, this time a lot more forcefully.

But then he gave another almighty tug and that's when the baby came out – but, oh my gosh, she looked so poorly! After five pulls, the poor thing was covered in cuts and bruises. To me, it was a clear case of medical negligence. Why had the registrar attempted the forceps with the baby so high in the pelvis? She could have had a C-section. But of course, nobody said a thing, the woman accepted her baby the way she came out (because she didn't know any different), and there were no consequences for the doctor. I guess they just aren't as expendable as midwives.

Don't get me wrong: I get on well with all the doctors on our ward. I respect them and we work well as a team, but you rarely hear of them being reprimanded or disciplined. Sam's experience had shown me that we couldn't rely on the hospital for support. Because while hierarchy and power flowed one way in our hospital, responsibility and blame flowed the other. It always seemed to be that if anything went wrong those of us on the bottom rung of the ladder were blamed first, because the consequences of blaming others higher up the food chain were more serious, and potentially more damaging to the hospital trust.

16

Could You Just . . .?

'*D*eck the halls with boughs of holly, fa la la la la la la la la la!*' I sang to Bev on reception desk.

"*'Tis the season to be jolly, fa la la la la la la la la!*' she sang back, and we both started to laugh. It was Christmas Eve and I was beyond excited. Tomorrow I would be spending my very first Christmas Day with Betty, and now that she was four years old she finally understood what all the fuss was about. At last! I felt like I'd waited for this moment for *years*.

I loved Christmas, I loved everything about it. The food, the tree, the presents – oh, especially the presents! I had started my Christmas present shopping back in September, and I'd built up a huge pile of gifts under our enormous tree.

'Don't you think that's enough?' Will asked one night, when he caught me sliding another pile of presents for Betty under the boughs, heavy with sparkly adornments.

'Oh, they're only a few little bits,' I said. 'Just some stocking-fillers.'

I hugged myself as I imagined her unwrapping all her

gifts in the morning. I looked at my watch – 2.45 a.m. She'd be in bed now, all tucked up, dreaming of Father Christmas and his magical reindeer. Earlier that day, Betty and I had sprinkled 'reindeer food' in the garden for Dasher, Dancer, Prancer, Vixen and Rudolph. It was adorable – she'd come home from nursery with the glittery pack of muesli, all wrapped up with a red and white ribbon and a laminated card attached with the poem: 'Just sprinkle on your lawn at night. The moon will make it sparkle bright. As Santa's reindeer fly and roam, this will guide them to your home'.

Now the tiny patch of grass outside the house was full of glitter and bits of raisin and oats, but I didn't care – she had loved throwing the stuff around, totally enchanted by the idea of feeding flying deer. In a fit of utter madness, my lovely (and very brave) Will had even offered to cook Christmas dinner for the whole family: his parents and mine. I imagined him in the kitchen, getting to work on the long list he'd set himself: peeling spuds, scoring the Brussels sprouts and stuffing the turkey. All, no doubt, helped by a large glass of something cold and alcoholic in his hand. I felt all warm and festive at the thought.

I readjusted the little red Rudolph clips in my hair. In the past couple of weeks, we'd all started wearing seasonal jewellery and hairpieces. I don't think any of us would have gone so far out of our way to look this festive, but it was more a show of solidarity for Katie, my student midwife, than anything else. She had been given a tongue-lashing by Lina for wearing a cute headband with antler deely-boppers.

'Those . . .' she'd said disdainfully, pointing to Katie's headwear, 'are not appropriate for work. Take them off. Now!' It was horrible and humiliating for Katie who, after all, was only trying to spread a little Christmas cheer on the ward. What was wrong with that? Lina was such a misery-guts – a real *Scrooge*.

The next day, the rest of us came in sporting Christmas earrings and hair adornments to show Lina just what we thought of her 'appropriate for work' rule. We went all out, buying Santa hats, glitterball headbands, Christmas pudding earrings and snowman necklaces. They weren't subtle in the least, but they were jolly, morale-boosting and fun. Best of all, I could tell that Lina didn't like them one bit – but she didn't have the bottle to give us a dressing down because we were all more senior than Katie. *A typical bully*, I thought, *picking on the ones she thought were too weak to fight back.*

At least she wasn't on tonight – no, it was a lovely group of midwives on this evening and every single woman was full to bursting with Christmas cheer. I kept breaking into carol-singing, and whoever was near me usually joined in. Instinctively, I checked my watch again: 2.52 a.m. *Just another four hours and eight minutes and I could go home!* In previous years, I'd volunteered to work the Christmas Day shift, because it was good pay, and I was happy to give the time off to my colleagues who had kids. But I felt that this year was *my* year. It was *my* time to start making those special family memories.

Mum had finally accepted that my relationship with Will was for keeps, and she and my dad were terrific hands-on grandparents to our daughter. I got on well with Will's folks too, who were also wonderful grandparents, and now I was looking forward to doing a proper Christmas with all the relatives round at ours for festive food, family games and fights over who was going to wash up.

I collected my paperwork and went back into the room where I was looking after a lovely woman. She was on her third child and was managing very well on gas and air, crouching on all fours. She seemed to be doing really well all by herself, so I just left her to it. Dad was great – very supportive and receptive to her needs, so they barely needed me at all. It was just another half an hour and out popped their beautiful little boy, easy as you like. Dad cut the cord and Mum wept a few happy tears.

'He's our surprise Christmas gift!' Mum said, smiling through her tears. 'There's seven years between him and his brother. I didn't even know I was pregnant until I was nearly four months gone. To be honest, we never thought we'd have three.'

'Let alone one born on Christmas Day,' said Dad. 'I suppose the other kids are going to get more than they bargained for this Christmas.'

'Didn't Aidan want an X Box?' Mum laughed.

'He's not getting an X Box,' said Dad, cradling his newborn. 'Anyway, this one's better than an X Box.'

'Hmmm . . . I'm not sure Aidan's going to agree with you on that one,' Mum said, laughing. I gave them both a cup of tea and some toast and left the room to complete the paperwork. It was 5 a.m.– just enough time to get all the admin finished before the end of my shift.

I was sat in the staffroom, filling out the online pathway, registering the new NHS number, the centile growth chart, registering the birth and starting their postnatal notes when Lucy, the night-time coordinator, popped her head round the door.

'Ah, Pippa!' she exclaimed.

Could You Just . . .?

'Hiya, Lucy.' I looked up briefly from my papers.

'Just the person I wanted to see.' She grinned, walking towards me.

'Oh, really?' *Uh-oh. I don't like the sound of this.*

'Yes. Could you just come in to see this lady? It won't be hard; we might be going in for a section and I need an extra pair of hands.' I checked my watch again.

'It won't take long, I'm sure of it,' Lucy hurried on. 'She's thirty-four weeks but she's showing signs of infection and the baby's heart rate is quite flat, a bit unresponsive. I think they're going to be taking her into theatre pretty soon and I just need another midwife. Do you think . . .?'

'Yeah, sure,' I said, grinning. I knew there wasn't going to be a whole lot of spare midwives kicking around at 5 a.m. on Christmas Day – and, besides, I still had two hours before my shift ended.

By the time I got to the room and was fully briefed, the consultant was scrubbing up and Anna was being prepped to be taken to theatre. She was conscious and talking to her husband Pete. Though naturally anxious, they were both calm and he held her hand as she was wheeled down to theatre. I wasn't surprised – their main midwife was a very experienced older lady called Jill. She was a very soothing presence, and I knew they would have first-class care from her.

The consultant and registrar conducted the section together. In no time at all the baby was out, and everyone was relieved that she seemed perfectly healthy. We took her measurements, wrapped her in a towel, and I was just about to hand her to the mum, Anna, when she started to bleed. It was one of those occasions where the whole place seemed to be covered in deep-claret blood in a matter of moments. It poured off the table and pooled onto the floor.

'To the dad,' the consultant muttered, and so I swerved, changing direction to hand the baby immediately to Pete instead of Anna. 'She's haemorrhaging.'

The team was quick to act, calling in the appropriate people, putting calls out for Obstetric Emergency, arranging blood from the Blood Bank, weighing and estimating blood loss.

'Can we get the dad out now, please,' urged the consultant.

'BP seventy-forty, unstable,' called out the anaesthetist. 'Heart rate a hundred and twenty increasing, saturation good, oxytocin having no effect. Starting propofol for the GA. Stand clear of the head, please, so I can intubate.'

'Someone alert Blood Bank,' said the consultant. 'Possible major haemorrhage protocol to follow. Can people stand clear of the head, please!' Now the anaesthetist inserted the airway. 'Intubation and ventilation complete, Misoprostol and coags administered, transfusion current and stable. She's all yours.'

We all knew this was serious. Anna had been given a general anaesthetic and Pete was ushered out of the room to the birthing suite, as the consultant, Dr Thurgood, tried to get the bleeding under control. He had already completed surgery and finished suturing the abdomen, so he now tried to locate the bleed vaginally, looking for any trauma that needed suturing, requesting more oxytocin and coagulants to manage the bleeding. I checked the placenta to rule out any retained products that could cause bleeding, while the anaesthetist took more blood samples to check the clotting factors in the blood. By the time the bleeding had stopped, Anna had lost eight litres of blood.

Could You Just . . .?

Dr Thurgood inserted a Bakri balloon, which inflates with water to put pressure on the inside of the uterine wall to stop any further bleeding. Anna was transferred down to ITU. It was 6 a.m. when we emerged from theatre, all of us shaken by what had just happened. And I still had another two hours of paperwork from the earlier birth to complete before I could leave. *So much for getting out of here on time*, I thought. I cursed Lucy. *So much for 'it won't take long'.*

This time I perched myself on the reception desk to get the rest of my paperwork completed while Dr Thurgood did his own papers next to me. We worked quietly side by side as the sun came up on Christmas morning – until at 7.30 a.m., the ringing of the phone made us both jump. I picked up.

'Hi, this is Pam from the ITU team. Your caesarean lady here has lost another two and half litres and the Bakri isn't working. We're going to have to take her back into theatre.'

I put my hand over the receiver and spoke to Dr Thurgood: 'She's lost another two and a half litres.'

He gestured for me to pass the phone over and then he spoke to her: 'Okay, let's take her back to theatre. I will meet you in there. I'm coming over now.' Then he passed the phone back to me and shot off down the corridor.

'Is the husband there?' Pam asked.

'No, he's gone home to take care of the other kids,' I replied.

'Well, you probably could do with giving him a call and getting him back here. In all honesty, it doesn't look too good. She's on her way down to main theatre as we speak, and if we can't stabilise her and stop this bleed, well . . . we're running out of options.'

209

'Okay. I'll do that now.' I put down the phone and the reality of the situation suddenly hit me. Anna's life was in the balance. She could die at any moment and I had to tell her husband. The ringtone at the other end of the phone blared loudly in my ears as I waited for Peter to pick up, my heart beating faster with every ring. After a handful of rings, there was a click and his voice came on the line:

'Hello?'

'Peter, it's Pippa George, one of the midwives at the hospital.'

'Oh hi. Everything alright?' I could hear the joyful squeals of children unwrapping presents in the background. Peter now shouted: 'Kids! Kids! Hush. Be quiet. It's the hospital on the phone.' Then he addressed me: 'Sorry about that, Pippa, they're so excited, what with Christmas and a new baby, it's a mad house! Anyway, what can I do you for?'

'Peter, Anna has lost more blood in ITU, so they're taking her back to theatre straightaway. We think . . .' my voice started to crack. 'We think you better come back to hospital as we are greatly concerned.'

There was a moment of shocked silence, followed by a quiet, 'I'm on my way. Thank you.' The line clicked as the phone rang off. By now, Lucy was by my side.

'Pippa, the daytime staff are here now. Your shift ended an hour and a half ago. You can go home now.'

'Erm . . . yeah, okay. It's Anna – she's gone back into theatre from ITU. Will you call me if you hear? Let me know?' I asked in a small voice.

'Yeah, sure. Now go on, go home. It's Christmas!'

* * *

Could You Just . . .?

I don't remember driving home that morning. One minute I turned on the engine in the car park of the hospital, the next I was pulling onto our drive. I must have been in a state of shock. Making that call to Peter had been one of the worst moments of my life. Having to tell a father who, only moments before, had been enjoying Christmas with his children, that he could be losing his wife was horrific. And even now I didn't know if she was alive or dead. I was in a complete daze. Nothing seemed quite real. Will was already up with Betty, the pair of them fizzing with energy and excitement and, remarkably, he'd managed to stop her opening any of her gifts without me. But I could barely speak.

'You okay?' he mouthed at me as Betty bounced up and down on the sofa, gripping a large oblong present, begging me to let her open it.

'Please can I? Please, please, please, please,' she begged.

'Tell you later,' I mouthed back, then, 'Go on,' I said, smiling at Betty. 'You can open it.'

I don't remember what happened next. I'd like to say that our first Christmas morning together as a family was every bit as magical as I'd imagined, but I can't recall any of it. I was absent. I may have talked, smiled and joked while I played with Betty, but really I was just going through the motions, not taking any of it in.

My strongest memory of that day, of that first special family Christmas I'd planned so hard for, was of lying on my bed upstairs, sobbing uncontrollably. I just couldn't stop thinking of Anna and Peter. How could I possibly enjoy Christmas knowing what that family was going through? My own family arrived at the house, Will's family too. Everyone made a big fuss of Betty and I managed to blend

211

into the background, unable to enjoy all the fun around me. Will cooked an amazing lunch, which I could only pick at, and in the afternoon I managed to get my head down and sleep for a few hours. At 6 p.m., when I woke up, Will said I'd missed a call from the hospital. I called them straight back. Sam was on shift and she gave me the news.

In all, Anna had lost sixteen litres of blood, around three times the amount we have in our bodies. They couldn't get the blood into her quick enough before it came straight out again. They had finally stabilised her at around midday, and then she'd been airlifted to a bigger hospital where she was going to go for embolization (where a catheter is inserted into an artery in the groin and guided under xray to place embolic agents – such as tiny bits of plastic the size of grains of sand, or small fragments of medical sponge – to stop further bleeding). It was still touch and go, but she was alive and stable at least. Will hugged me after I put the phone down.

'I'm sorry,' I wept in his arms. 'This wasn't how it was meant to be.'

'It's okay, don't worry,' he whispered, stroking my hair. 'Betty didn't notice a thing. She's had a lovely day.'

'Really?' I welled up again.

'Yeah. You picked some great presents. She loves them. Of course she thinks Santa brought them all, so you won't be getting any credit but, hey, that's the magic bit, right?'

'You're brilliant, thank you.' I grinned. If it hadn't been for Will, the whole of Christmas would have fallen apart.

'I burnt the potatoes and ruined a pan,' he said.

'I didn't notice,' I laughed.

'That's why I love you.'

17

All in the Mind

W hy is it always the mums with a needle phobia who need the most injections? I have to say that, in my many years of midwifery, it seems to be a painful truth that if you've got a fear of needles – or trypanophobia, to give it its official name – you're most likely to end up getting pricked like a pin cushion! They are *always* the ones who need the blood tests, extra drugs and pain relief. And I know it's mischievous, but I do find it amusing when a mum comes in covered in extravagant tattoos and tells me she can't stand needles.

'What? With all this beautiful artwork?' I say with a smile.

Then there is tokophobia, a phobia of giving birth itself – now that's a strange one. Most women feel a certain trepidation and nervousness about the birth – after all, there are few things harder than trying to push a baby out of your vagina – but a real phobia of giving birth is utterly paralysing. In these cases, the woman will usually be given a C-section, unless she has already gone into labour, in which case we just have to keep her as calm as possible through different breathing techniques, aromatherapy, music and generally trying to be as reassuring as possible.

Mental wellbeing is something we are always aware of, particularly after the birth itself. Every woman experiences a different set of circumstances leading up to the birth with, for example, their family situation, the state of their relationship, previous mental health issues and underlying stresses that may manifest in serious ways after the baby is born, even to the point of psychosis. Then labour itself is one of the most stressful things both body and mind can go through – and it is quite natural that some mothers feel detached at first. The ones that have been through a serious physical trauma don't always experience that instant 'rush of love' within the first twenty-four hours. It takes them a little time to get over the physical and mental aspect of birth, which is perfectly normal, and understandable of course, though they beat themselves up about it because they expect to be overwhelmed with love. Instead they are overwhelmed with pain, exhaustion and shock. Perhaps in today's society, we have an idealised notion of how motherhood should look and feel, which results in new mothers being surprised by their own emotions – or rather, lack of them.

'When will I feel this big surge of love everyone talks about?' I get asked quite often. Detachment is much more common than people realise, so we always encourage new mums to bond with their baby by spending time with them, holding them, and having as much skin-to-skin contact as possible.

Bonding can be a particular concern for babies born of rape victims. Because of the circumstances of how they were conceived, we are aware that these mums can experience mixed feelings towards their babies. And yet, in one rape case I dealt with, it wasn't the mother who had problems with the baby – it was her family. Kayla's was a truly shocking story. The last thing this young, twenty-year-old woman recalled was walking home after a drunken night out with her friends. Next, she was waking up in a side street, clothes hanging off, aware that she felt something may have happened *down below* but she couldn't be sure because she didn't remember a thing. Luckily, she had the presence of mind to take herself straight to A&E, where the rape was confirmed, and the police called. A trawl of CCTV film from that night in the town centre immediately identified a suspect, and in time he was arrested and charged.

'We didn't think it was a good idea to go ahead with the pregnancy,' her mother confided in the delivery suite. 'I mean, this child will be a daily reminder of what happened. We just thought it would be best if she moved on with . . .'

'My child is innocent,' Kayla interrupted her mother. 'And if anything good can come out of what happened then I think that's a positive thing.' Her mother clamped her mouth shut and gave me a look that said: 'See!'

'Besides, he's in prison now and he's never going to have anything to do with her, Social Services have assured me,' Kayla went on. She had coped very well with the labour so far, and I could tell she was a strong character.

'Oh well, she's made her mind up now,' the mother sighed. 'It's too late to do anything about it. All we can do is support her and give her all the help she needs.'

Kayla wasn't in a relationship, so her mum was her birthing partner, and she would need all her family's support over the next few months. Thankfully, the delivery was fairly straightforward, and once the little girl was born, all the mixed feelings in the room were replaced with joy and delight. Kayla seemed besotted with her baby from the word go. I just hoped that once the initial euphoria had worn off and Kayla was at home with her little girl, her feelings remained positive.

* * *

It is rare to see a serious case of psychosis; however, we do come across it occasionally. We had one woman who wouldn't look at her baby, she just kept muttering to herself, sitting on the side of the bed, rocking and rubbing her knees. That's all she did, all night long. She didn't get an ounce of sleep and didn't attend to her baby's needs in any way. In the morning, we brought in the psychiatric team, who confirmed that they also had concerns with the new mum's behaviour and thinking process, so plans were made that when she was discharged from our maternity care she would go straight to one of the psychiatric mother and baby units. But it is unusual to see that happen so quickly after birth. Post-natal depression (PND) doesn't usually manifest straight away – most cases of PND come on after the mums have left our ward, so it is not something I see often. If there is a history of PND often there will be a care plan in place. Underlying mental health issues are usually known about before the pregnancy or are picked up by the community midwife. In some extreme cases, we see behaviour that no one could possibly class as normal – and in these instances, it's very hard to rationalise the mother's actions. Our role as the midwife ends when the baby is born, and the community and psychiatric teams take over if necessary, so we don't have anything more to do with the mothers. I often wonder about them and just hope they're OK.

One day, I was called over to the nurses' station after Jen took a call at Reception.

'Right, we might need some extra support with this one,' she said to the assembled team. 'An ambulance is on its way, bringing in a young female who has just given birth and is bleeding vaginally. Ambulance Control, who have been liaising with the police, have told me that our lady has given the name Olga and works in a food-packing factory. At around 10.30 this morning, a colleague, one of the factory workers, went to the toilet. There, they heard an unusual sound coming from one of the cubicles. She went to investigate and found what looked like a full-term baby lying feet first down the toilet. Obviously, she pulled the baby out and raised the alarm immediately. Subsequently, it appears the mother was discovered at her work station, bleeding heavily through her jeans.

'When questioned by the police, Olga claimed she didn't know she was pregnant until the baby was born, and appears to be in a state of shock. The baby is stable and is en route via air ambulance to the neonatal intensive care unit, but Olga is coming to us. As far as we're aware, after a quick check of the system, she hasn't booked in with any midwife or confirmed the pregnancy with a GP.'

Olga arrived on our unit fifteen minutes later – she was small, tiny in fact, slim, and appeared to be in her early twenties. She looked very young, I thought, and I could imagine that if she had known she was pregnant, she could easily have concealed the bump under baggy clothes.

Post-partum, you couldn't tell at all that she had just given birth. She also wore the expression of a deer caught in headlights. She looked terrified as we showed her into a private room so the doctor could assess her and check if the placenta was still inside and try to estimate blood loss. Afterwards, we settled her on the ward. According to the neonatal unit, the baby boy had an infection, but he seemed otherwise healthy. I was assigned to look after Olga, and when I joined her on the ward I did my best to put her at her ease.

'Hello, Olga. I'm Pippa. I'm the midwife who will be looking after you today. How are you feeling?'

She shrugged. She seemed frightened and refused to make eye contact.

'I see here it says you're originally from Poland,' I went on. 'We've had a look for you on our system but we haven't found anything. Have you got a doctor here in the UK?'

'No, no doctor.'

'Right, so you didn't see a doctor about the pregnancy? No blood tests? Scans? Nothing?'

'I didn't know about baby,' she said quietly. 'It was shock.'

'Okay, okay, sweetheart, that's fine. I tell you what, why don't I get you a nice cup of tea or a coffee and a few biscuits and you can tell me what happened?'

There was a long pause, and then Olga, eyes full of tears, sighed and looked up at the ceiling.

'I go to work and suddenly I feel big pain in stomach, so I go to toilet and then . . . *urgh* . . . it was just great pain. And blood. And then, I don't realise – baby come out. I don't know . . . I don't know. After that, I am getting scared. I don't know what to do. I must go back to work or they don't pay me and I lose job, so I go back to my work. But then, there is blood. Lots of blood, and then police and ambulance come and bring me hospital. And that is it.'

'Okay. Are you married? Do you have a boyfriend, Olga?' I asked. 'Is there a partner we should contact about the birth?'

'No, no boyfriend,' she whispered.

'Olga, do you know who the father is?' She shook her head. She still wouldn't look me in the eyes.

'I live in big house,' she said. 'There are many, many Polish workers in the house. Many men. I . . . I don't know who father is . . .' she tailed off and refused to say any more. She seemed ashamed and I wondered if she really was twenty-three, as it said on her notes, or far younger.

I scanned the report from the police – they had discovered a pair of box cutters in the toilet cubicle where the baby was found.

'The box cutters?' I asked. 'What were they used for?'

'There was rope in me. I use it for the rope to the baby.'

She used box cutters to cut the cord? Wow.

'Am I in trouble?' she asked now in a small voice. 'Will I go prison?'

I was stunned – she didn't ask how her baby was; she didn't seem to care at all about the young life she had left for dead in a toilet. No, the only thing she cared about was getting into trouble. I didn't know how to reply.

'Why don't you rest, love?' I suggested. 'I think the police are going to want to speak to you again soon about what happened. You'll just have to tell them the truth.'

Perhaps she *was* in shock. Perhaps the trauma of the birth meant she'd temporarily lost her mind, making her prioritise her work commitments over the life of her child.

But to me the whole thing was incomprehensible. Was she really living and working under gulag conditions where she was afraid to miss time out of her shift to give birth? The factory she worked for wasn't exactly a beacon of workers' rights – still, I couldn't quite square it. Olga was arrested but, in the end, the police decided against prosecution and, thankfully, the baby survived its horrific start in life and was placed into the custody of the local authority, to go onto permanent adoption, which was Olga's choice.

But something bothered me about that case. I did wonder about Olga's story. I know people do strange things when they are in shock, but when she saw the baby, she didn't scream or cry out for help, she just put the toilet seat down and walked away. If she had no idea she was pregnant, wouldn't the arrival of the baby have caused her to scream? Raise the alarm? Get help? But she hadn't done any of those things. She had picked up a pair of box cutters, cut the cord, abandoned the baby down the toilet and then walked away. Had she temporarily lost her mind or were her personal circumstances so desperate she couldn't possibly fathom bringing a baby into the world? I just couldn't work it out.

* * *

But it was the case of sepsis that threw me for six. I had assisted a woman called Deborah in the vaginal delivery of her first child, a little girl, and everything had seemed absolutely fine after the birth, so she was discharged home. However, she was admitted back onto the ward two weeks later, shivering, with a high temperature. She obviously had an infection of some kind, perhaps caused by some placenta remaining inside her. She said she'd passed a few clots, so the doctors took her into theatre for a manual removal, just to ensure there wasn't any placenta left behind. That would allow the uterus to contract down properly.

I cared for Deborah and recovered her from theatre after she came back out, taking her observations every five minutes. But from the start, the figures were all over the place. Her blood pressure was up and down, temperature swinging from high to low, and her pulse was getting faster and faster. After fifteen minutes of this confusing picture, I called the anaesthetist back in.

'What's happening?' I asked. 'I can't make head nor tail–'

'Oh shit, she's septic,' the anaesthetist said. He pressed the emergency buzzer straight away and, as people started to pile into the room, he spoke quickly: 'Okay, this lady is now becoming septic. I need a few hands to help cannulate, put in fluids and commence antibiotics.'

But before he got a chance to finish his sentence, Deborah's eyes widened and she sat bold upright, demanding: 'WHO ARE YOU? WHAT DO YOU WANT?'

'Deborah, this is Dr Abay, he's the anaesthetist who–'

'GET OFF! GET OFF ME! WHO ARE YOU? WHO ARE THESE PEOPLE? GET ME OUT OF HERE!'

Deborah's partner Luke was also in the room, holding their two-week-old infant in his arms. He got up to try to reassure his wife. 'Deborah! They're trying to help. Dr Abay. Pippa. You remember? She's our midwife. They're trying to help you. Please just calm down.'

But it was no use. Deborah was in septic shock – she was delirious and the sudden appearance of all these strange faces alarmed her further. She didn't know where she was or who we were. Her eyes were full of fear now, and as the various members of the team tried to get hold of her arms to administer fluids and antibiotics, she whipped them away, ripping her skin as she tore at the cannulas. In her delirium, she couldn't see that we were trying to make her well again. She was petrified, thinking we were attacking her, and started to fight us off. Now Deborah tried to climb off the bed, but she'd had a spinal for the operation, so she was numb from the waist down.

'Hold her down!' the registrar shouted, and six pairs of hands immediately clamped down on her arms and shoulders. Her legs were useless; if she'd managed to get off the bed she would have just fallen on the floor.

'NOOOOOO!' Deborah roared like a wounded animal.

Everyone leaped into action. I put myself on the scribe roll, writing down everyone who was in the room, what was happening and who was putting what drugs into her, while the obstetrics team decided how best to manage her. Meanwhile, Deborah was completely out of control.

'YOU BASTARDS! GET OFF ME. GET BACK. DON'T TOUCH ME! *ARRGHGH!*' she screamed and struggled against the medics. It was very distressing, as well as chaotic and stressful. Remaining calm and focused was the only answer. I had to stay on top of the scribe, knowing that if I missed one vital piece of information it could cost this woman her life.

'Tazocin going in.'

'Second litre of hartmanns up and running.'

'Observations are still all over the place.'

'BP dropping, temp rising.'

'PV loss moderate, not excessive, no clots.'

All in the Mind

'Can someone inform Critical Care and ask them to review, please? She needs to be transferred to ITU.'

It was hard to keep on top of it all because lots of people were doing lots of different things at the same time to stabilise the situation, but the team worked well together. Deborah fought us like a wild tigress, but eventually we got a cannula into her and she was sedated, stabilised and given antibiotics.

'I jussss . . . don't . . . *nnnnnggg* . . . ' Her speech slowed right down and became slurred until she flopped back onto the bed. It took another forty-five minutes before we could stabilise her properly and then she was taken to ITU to recover. The worst over, we all staggered out of that room like shell-shocked soldiers. I'd honestly never seen anything like it in my entire life.

For the next two days, I was constantly on the phone to ITU, checking on Deborah, making sure she was okay. Slowly, but surely, she recovered. Meanwhile, the team tried to analyse what had happened. According to the consultant, if there was infected tissue left behind after the birth, the manual evacuation could have actually made things worse, pushing it into her blood stream. Two days later, the infection now in retreat, Deborah returned to our ward and I was relieved to find she was her normal self again.

I went into her room and she smiled blandly at me.

'How you feeling, Deborah?' I asked.

'Hmmm . . . okay, I suppose.' There was an unmistakable blankness in her eyes. She didn't recognise me.

'Do you know who I am?' I asked.

'I'm sorry. You seem familiar, but I'm really not sure why.'

'It's Pippa. Pippa George. You really don't remember me? I delivered your baby two weeks ago.'

'Yeah, it's just I had an infection and I don't really remember anything about the birth.'

'I know,' I said gently. 'I was there. You tried to bite my face.'

Though Deborah's delirium had a clear physical cause, we always have to be aware of mental health issues surrounding birth. After all, it is probably the most stressful time in a woman's life. People often think about the physical trauma of going through the process of labour, but in fact the mental one can be just as harmful – we tend to forget that giving birth is an assault on a woman's identity and status. So much is compromised: a woman's privacy, her dignity and even her identity as an autonomous individual making her own choices in the world. It's not the same for everyone – for some women the process is wonderful, they have a terrific experience and nothing but good memories of the birth. But for others, from the moment they go into labour all their previous notions of personhood slip away. And after all of that, you have a baby to look after who is 100 per cent dependent on you. It can be brutal. No wonder we have to be watchful of mental health in these circumstances. Mental wellbeing is a crucial part of the birthing process and we can't afford to take it for granted.

18

Sink or Swim?

It's not just the expectant mums that I'm watching out for, sometimes it's the dads I need to keep my eye on. A dad fainted on me once. I was looking after first-time mum Maya in a birthing pool and her partner Julian was gently propped over the side. She had warned me earlier that Julian was 'a bit squeamish', and he had nodded in agreement.

'No problem.' I'd smiled at them both. 'Julian, why don't you sit behind your wife and that way all you'll be able to see is her and the baby when she arrives? You won't see any of the other stuff.'

They both did very well with this arrangement, and he held her hand tightly, stopping Maya from dipping below the surface whenever she let go of the pool's edge. She delivered the baby beautifully all by herself and then pulled him up to her chest. I had been sat behind her, monitoring the birth, when suddenly I felt a heavy weight on my shoulder – it was Julian, slumped and unconscious, sliding down the edge of the pool. I gently laid him down on the floor and went to fetch some water while my student dealt with Maya.

Pool births are my favourite. People imagine all sorts of things, but a hospital birthing pool is like a very deep bath. Once it's full, the mum can sit vertically in the warm water for most of the birth and can often manage her pain better, taking in just gas and air as she needs it, and usually progresses well in this way. And here, I'll let you in on a little secret: nine times out of ten, a woman will poo in labour. Really, it shouldn't be a secret at all. I mean, it's natural and completely predictable – after all, all that pressure on that one area of the body makes some sort of evacuation fairly inevitable. And yet, of all the bodily functions that take place in labour, it is the one thing ALL women get embarrassed about. Fortunately, I have a little sieve for just such purposes.

'Oh no! Have I shit myself?' they might ask, alarmed.

'No, no,' I lie, scooping up the little brown floaters behind her back.

'Are you sure? I can smell poo.'

'No, that's nothing. Now keep pushing!'

By the end, I'm usually soaked from head to foot, with dripping wet hair. Or sporting two large round wet patches on my uniform where I've leaned forward and dipped my boobs into the water (not a good look). And we have a healthy newborn baby! It's the aftermath when things can go awry. It's not just dads; I've had women faint in the pool, almost bleed out and all sorts!

A couple of years ago, I had a lady who had given birth beautifully but then, as she pulled the baby up to her, the cord snapped around her vagina in the pool. But because it was under the water, nobody noticed. All I could see was that there was bleeding in the pool and assumed it was from the mother. It wasn't until the baby started to go pale and floppy that I realised there was something wrong. That's when I saw the cord had snapped and the baby was haemorrhaging. Once we got a clamp on the cord the baby instantly revived, but she remained very pale. Babies don't have much blood to lose, and I was furious with myself for not recognising the problem sooner. The paediatrician reviewed the baby but, thankfully, her iron levels were okay and, after a few days of being on the neonatal unit and monitoring increasing iron levels, she didn't need a transfusion.

Once a baby is born in a birthing pool, it is then a team effort to get mum and baby out of the pool as quickly and safely as we can. Then you're left with a pool full of afterbirth, blood, poo and all sorts of bodily fluids. It's the women's choice where and how they deliver the placenta. In my experience, women mostly let it come naturally in the pool after a few position changes and slight maternal effort, so with all that extra stuff there's no question – it can get a bit yucky in the pool after a birth.

Generally, with pool births, I like to stay hands off and let the mother do it on her own. I'll only get involved if there's a complication. The thing is, you can never quite predict what's going to happen in labour. You can have a run of smooth births where everything is nice and normal, and the next week you could be hit with forceps, third-degree tears, haemorrhages, shoulder dystocia – the lot! Shoulder dystocia is one you don't want to see, especially not in the pool. That's when the head comes out fine, but the baby's shoulders get wedged and the baby becomes stuck. At this point you've got a maximum of seven minutes to get the baby out before it is compromised, so the clock is ticking. There are a few things you can do – and trust me, I've done all of them, including getting in the pool myself – but a good manoeuvre is to get the lady to put one leg up on the side of the pool. Sometimes just that movement of bringing one leg right up is enough to release the baby's impacted shoulder.

Then, as soon as the baby is out, I transform from midwife into photographer extraordinaire! It's a bit like Superman's quick change in the telephone box – only slightly less dramatic. I whip off my blood-covered gloves, grab the mum's phone, call for 'Smiles' and then take that precious first picture of the just-born baby with their slightly stunned and emotional parents. Luckily, I've managed to avoid dropping any expensive iPhones into the pool (so far!), though quite a few of my pens have gone under water. Babies change so quickly, especially in the first few days after birth, so it's really important to record that first moment they arrive in the world.

'Smile!'

Snap!

'Smile!'

Snap!

Then it's another quick change, gloves back on, in time to deliver the placenta. We occasionally get requests from dads to film the birth, but in our hospital there is a 'no filming' policy, which I can understand. Suppose the video gets into the wrong hands or someone puts it online without getting the woman's consent? In my view, the rule is there for a reason – which is not to say that some midwives won't bend the rules. It all depends who you get on the day.

Generally, the dads that come onto our ward make pretty

good birthing partners. In the run up to the birth, many have usually attended a couple of antenatal sessions or even a course of NCT (Natural Childbirth Trust) classes, so they know what to expect. And even if they're not particularly hands on, most are keen to be involved in some way. It's rare to come across a dad that doesn't rise to the occasion, but they do exist. In my early years, while I was still training, we had one dad who just sat in the corner of the delivery room reading a book, completely ignoring his wife, who was trying to push his baby through her vagina. I found it infuriating. I kept looking at Bev, eyebrows raised, as if to say: *Is this guy for real?* Eventually, Bev went straight up to him and literally plucked the book out of his hands.

'You really need to be here for her at this stage,' she said sternly, placing the book safely out of his reach. It didn't help much. After Bev's intervention, he just sat there holding his wife's hand, looking away, as if this was the most boring thing in the world. It was better when he was reading the book. We were bringing new life into the world, for goodness sake! I just didn't understand his indifference. *Why are you even here?* I wondered. *And how on earth does she put up with it?* I would have sent him packing.

Occasionally, a drunk dad pitches up on the ward, though not always by design. One father-to-be had been out on the town with his mates for a stag do when his wife went into labour unexpectedly. He rolled onto the ward, merry, loud and full of good cheer. It was quite amusing from our point of view – he was like a footie fan cheering from the stands for his favourite team: 'Yeah, come on, Mel!' he yelled enthusiastically. 'You can do it! Come on, gal!'

But Mel wasn't amused. In fact, Mel was really miffed.

'Oh, shut up, Fin,' she snapped. 'You're drunk.'

'Juusss giving you some mortal support,' he slurred.

'You mean *moral* support,' she sighed.

'Yup, that's the one . . . *moral support.*'

'Well, don't,' she said, 'it's annoying.'

By the end of that birth, mortal *was* the right word. I think she wanted to kill him.

To my mind, it's just as important to look after the dads as the birthing mother. After all, this is all new to them too, and they need just as much reassurance and handholding. Sometimes more than the women. I like the phone calls when the dads ring and you can hear the utter panic in their voices.

'*Arghhh!* Things are starting. It's all a bit much so we're coming in.'

'Okay, just calm down. Tell me what's happening . . . how frequent are the contractions?'

I try to get them to relax, take a few deep breaths and engage them in a little conversation.

'And how are you? Are you alright? Now look, everything that's happening is *normal.* I think you need to have a bit of a breather. Make yourself a cup of tea and make your partner one.'

A little reassurance can go a long way. It's their experience as well, even though they're not going through the labour. You want it to be okay for them, not horrified by it all, so I have to keep repeating – it's normal, everything's normal, don't worry. By the end, I sound like a broken record, but as long as it's enough to reassure them and keep them calm then it doesn't matter.

Even when you're in the delivery suite and things aren't

going quite according to plan, I may be busy with the emergency in hand, but I'll always engage the dad with eye contact, mouthing the words: 'It's all right. I'll talk to you in a bit'.

It's important to keep them fully informed throughout. Then, if we're going into theatre, I hand them some scrubs to change into in the toilets, and afterwards I like to give them a job, something to do to help. It makes them feel useful. I'll call them over and point to a monitor: 'Will you do me a really big favour and push this through for me?'

Once in the theatre, they're sat at their partner's head and their only role is to look after the mother, which can be hard because they have to appear calm and relaxed even though they might be feeling the exact opposite inside.

While I was sat on the nurses' desk, writing up all the paperwork from the 'fainting dad' pool birth, I took a panicked call from a partner during a home delivery. The community midwife hadn't arrived, and labour had progressed too quickly to get to hospital, so the dad, Jason, had to do it all himself. By the time he came through to me, he had already worked himself up into a real lather.

'I can see something, it's coming, it's coming,' he babbled down the phone.

'Okay, Jason,' I said, in what I hoped was my most reassuring voice. 'The most important thing now is to stay calm because your wife needs you to be on top of this. Don't worry – I'll stay with you on the line. My name is Pippa. Where is your wife now?'

'Nadia's in the middle of the lounge and she's definitely pushing.'

'Good. That's fine. Everything's fine.'

'I don't know what's happened to our community midwife, Pippa. We called her half an hour ago but no one's here. I mean, we thought she'd be here by now.'

'Don't worry. You can do this, Jason. We'll do it together. Now the first thing to do is to go and get some clean towels.'

The line fell silent as Jason dashed off on the towel mission. Now one of my colleagues sent for an ambulance while I waited for Jason to come back on the line. After about a minute . . .

'Okay, I've got the towels,' he panted breathlessly.

'Good. Just keep them close, as we'll need them to keep baby dry and warm later. Tell me, what can you see?'

'I can see the head. It's got hair! I can see it.'

'Okay, Jason, you're doing great. Just take a few breaths. How's Nadia doing?'

'Alright, alright, alright. You alright, love? Yeah, she's nodding. She's alright.' Then more waiting in silence.

'Put me on speakerphone so I can hear what's happening.'

Now I could hear his wife continuing to push, with the contractions coming every minute. They were good strong contractions lasting one minute.

'Right, Jason, we've sent an ambulance, and a community midwife will be there shortly. Is the front door unlocked so they can get in?' Then more waiting in silence, as Jason went to unlock the front door.

Eventually, he exploded: 'The baby's here. She's here! It's a girl! I'm a dad! I'm a fucking dad!'

Without realising it, I was holding my breath, waiting for that first cry. Waiting, waiting . . . just waiting. But I didn't hear anything, so I said, 'Jason, take the baby and dry her. It will stimulate her.'

Finally, the cry erupted, loud and strong. *Thank goodness!* I blinked back my own tears as I heard Jason and Nadia laughing and weeping down the line.

'Jason? Can you hear me, Jason? Put her on Nadia's chest,' I instructed. At that point, I heard the unmistakable wail of an ambulance siren on the line, growing louder and louder.

'It's here!' Jason shouted, now laughing and crying at the same time.

'Bloody hell, mate, you're too late,' he greeted the paramedic. 'She's out already! I've got a girl, pal, a little perfect girl she is!'

'Okay, Jason. You did brilliantly – you both did. Well done and congratulations. Now I'm going to have to go and leave you in their hands.'

'Thank you, Pippa.'

'You're most welcome,' I said, holding back my own tears of joy.

And then we hung up. I wondered if they would be brought onto the ward. That was always amazing, meeting a couple you'd talked through a home birth. But in the following few hours before the end of my shift, I didn't see Jason, Nadia and their new baby girl. This was a good sign – it meant everything was normal at home.

That day was all about phone calls. At around 6 p.m., an hour before my shift ended, I took a phone call from a man called Tony whose wife Gaynor was in labour. This was the second time Tony had called the ward during my shift. Now I spoke to Gaynor on the phone. I looked at my previous notes from the last call: *contractions were every seven minutes lasting thirty seconds, intact waters. Advice given: paracetamol, hot bath and reassurance, call back when contractions closer together.*

'Hi, Gaynor, my name's Pippa. How are you doing?

'It's painful. My contractions are now every five minutes, my waters still haven't gone, is that okay?'

'That's absolutely fine. How are you coping at home with the contractions? Did you take paracetamol and have a warm bath? Is your partner with you?'

'Yes, I did all the things they told me to do. I'm okay at home for now. Going to try going back in the bath, as that helped.'

'Okay, Gaynor, stay at home a little longer, but if there is any change or these contractions start coming more regular, then just call back. You have our number. Just remember to drink plenty of fluids and keep eating little and often.'

That was it. Our conversation ended, so I quickly made notes on the telephone sheet before answering another call, as the phone lines were crazy busy. Then it was handover time and my shift ended. Driving home in the early morning traffic, I thought about Jason and Nadia. The call from Tony went completely out of my mind. Little did I realise six months later that those two calls from Gaynor and Tony would come to take on a huge significance in my life.

19

Courting Trouble

'**D**o we want onion bhajis?' Will called out, as he ordered our Saturday night takeaway over the phone. We'd both had a heavy week and we were rewarding ourselves with an Indian takeaway. Since Betty arrived, we weren't exactly the party people we had been in our youth. Most of our Saturday nights were spent at home with a takeaway and a few episodes of *Narcos* on Netflix, cuddled up on the sofa until one or both of us conked out. It never took long. I was usually in my pyjamas by 10 p.m. on a Saturday night.

Onion bhajis? My stomach heaved with the memory.

'God, no!' I replied. I used to love them, but I hadn't been able to look at a bhaji for weeks now, not since a very unfortunate delivery that put me off the savoury Indian snacks for life.

Nisha was on her fourth baby and had been in labour for a couple of hours but didn't appear to be progressing quickly.

'Do you want a piece of toast?' I offered. 'Maybe a sandwich?'

Food can give you an energy burst and get everything moving quicker, so we always encourage our ladies to eat in the early stages of labour. Nisha screwed up her nose. She clearly didn't fancy a piece of toast.

'Indu!' she spoke to her sister, who was her birthing partner. 'Can you get me something please? You know what I like.' Half an hour later, Indu returned with a salad and a couple of onion bhajis, which Nisha hoovered up enthusiastically. It did the trick – she rapidly progressed and twenty-five minutes later she started to push. Now, not everyone knows this, but some people vomit with pain. As Nisha started to push, the pain brought all the food back up and she started to vomit – onion bhaji vomit! Oh God, the smell was horrendous. Normally, I've got a steel stomach and can cope with the most revolting sights and smells, but I have to admit onion bhaji sick was probably the most disgusting thing I'd smelled in all my life. It took all my willpower not to throw up, too! I vowed then and there never to touch another onion bhaji in my life.*

Betty was now in bed and Will and I were catching up with the news from our respective weeks at work over two large glasses of red wine. Since we were both juggling our jobs with the childcare, it was hard to carve out the time and energy to actually sit down, look one another in the eye and talk properly. Sometimes I wondered what Will actually looked like these days! It was hard enough staying on top of my work and mothering duties, let alone making time to gaze adoringly at the man I'd chosen as my life partner. For one thing, there was a whole raft of new guidelines to get to grips with on the ward, and now I brought Will up

* I did, if you were wondering, but not for another year!

to speed on the latest round of changes. With midwifery, the advice seems to change every month. One minute you're swaddling, then 'swaddling can kill', so that's out. Cot bumpers, which were at one time all the rage, are now out. Babies can't be put down on their tummies, but neither can you leave newborns on their backs too long or they might get flat heads. And on and on it goes. So many rules! No wonder new mums get stressed out.

I was way ahead of most new mothers in terms of 'baby knowledge' with Betty, but I'd never actually mothered my own child before. And the one thing I discovered from the start was that the rules don't always match the reality. I mean, Betty loved sleeping on her tummy! There were some nights she just wouldn't settle unless she was lying on her front. In the end, I just let her fall asleep on me because, one: I figured it was probably the safest way of letting her sleep like this. And two: I had to get some sleep myself in order to be a functioning person in the morning.

Our latest guidelines advised us to delay cord-clamping for a good five minutes after the baby had delivered, until all the blood had gone from the cord to the baby. When I first qualified, we were advised to cut the cord as soon as baby was born – within a minute or two. Clamps on, cord cut. Done. Now the guidelines advised waiting until it stopped pulsating, otherwise the baby could miss a large percentage of their blood volume, putting them at risk of anaemia. Delayed cord-clamping would increase the iron levels in the baby's blood, and increase their stem cell count, which would help with the baby's growth and immunity.

Personally, I thought the delay was a good idea. I had

done quite a lot of medical research into the cord, after the incident in the pool where the cord snapped and the baby nearly bled out. When a baby is first born, the placenta is still working and it's pulsing, pushing the blood back into baby – you can actually feel it. But once the baby has all the blood out of the cord it stops and goes clear. In a full cord you can see the veins are thick with blood, but when there's nothing left in the vessels it just stops. That's when the placenta detaches. It is estimated that thirty per cent of the baby's blood volume is held within the placenta, so the placenta will naturally run out of blood and then this is the best time to cut the cord. So allowing the baby to get the full blood volume from the cord makes sense.

Our hospital guidelines seem to change as often as trends among new parents. There used to be a lot of stem cell collection, it was very popular when I first qualified, but I haven't seen it in years now. And placenta collection sometimes pops up, too. It's still a matter of dispute, but some people believe that the placenta is very nutritious – rich in iron, apparently – and could help fight the onset of postnatal depression. We've heard some really strange stories of people throwing placenta parties, making placenta pies, or placenta paellas! But by far the weirdest use of the placenta I've come across personally was by a hippy couple I looked after. They were a really nice pair, but they took this placenta business seriously. The mum stayed in hospital recovering from the haemorrhage she'd had post birth, and the dad took the placenta home with him after the birth. Then, every morning, he came onto the ward with a shake in a Nutribullet glass, which he explained was a fruit smoothie – with added placenta blended in! And she drank them all. *Urgh* . . . it makes my stomach turn just thinking about it. I couldn't eat my own placenta. Just give me an iron tablet and be done with it . . . but each to their own.

The new craze is to send it off to be freeze-dried, ground up and then put into little pills. Freeze-dried placenta pills! One of our nurses did it – the company provided her with the container to put the placenta in, which she then sent off to have it capsulated. But there have been a couple of worrying stories about encapsulation: I mean, do you know if the person who has done it is scientifically trained? Has it been stored and dehydrated properly? How do you know if it is even your own placenta? In one case a mother and baby caught a bacterial infection from the mother taking placenta pills. I can't actually see a whole lot of scientific research to back up the claims of placenta consumption being any good for the mother, and some practitioners have warned against it as a source of potential infection. But it does appeal to some, and you never know what plans people may have, so I always ask after the birth: 'Are you keeping this, or should I throw it?'

That night, however, the main thing on my mind was the latest development in the ongoing case of Tony and Gaynor. Six months earlier, Gaynor came in to give birth to her second child. She'd been in labour for a long time and we'd spoken briefly on the phone before she came onto the ward. I could hardly remember the conversation now, and by the time she and her husband Tony arrived, I'd left for the day, so I had very little to do with the family. It was a sad case. Gaynor wasn't getting very far pushing so the registrar decided to give her a ventouse delivery in theatre.

Everything went smoothly but the baby was born with no signs of life, and no amount of resuscitation could bring her back. Naturally, the family demanded answers and a post-mortem revealed a tentorial tear in the brain, which meant that the baby would never have survived. But when did the tear happen? That was the crucial question. If it had happened naturally there was no case of negligence, but if the tear had been caused by the ventouse delivery, then the hospital was responsible.

At first, I didn't think too hard about this case – after all, I hadn't been on the ward during the birth, and I had never even set eyes on Gaynor or Tony. Fiona had been the midwife looking after them and naturally we talked about but it, but to my mind, I simply wasn't involved. The only contact I'd had with the family was during two telephone calls to the hospital before they came in. But on Friday, I got a call on my mobile.

'Tony and Gaynor's solicitor called me this week,' I explained to Will. 'She told me they are talking to absolutely everyone who had contact with the family in the run up to the birth.'

'How was it?'

'Well, I wasn't worried to begin with. As I explained, I wasn't there when she gave birth and I never even met her, so I didn't think my evidence was relevant. But still, this solicitor tore me to shreds. She said my paperwork had been 'shoddy', 'slapdash' and 'inadequate', and that really shocked me. I asked how she came to think that, and she said it was because I failed to put the date and time on top of one of the call sheets. And because of my 'careless record-keeping', I could be responsible for the baby's death.'

'What? That's ridiculous.'

'I know, I know. But still, it's making me doubt myself. I've since looked at my notes. I know that my advice to the woman was fine. Faultless. There was nothing wrong with what I told her. And I guess the solicitor agreed because she didn't take me up on my advice at all. The thing is, while I noted down her telephone number and address, I failed to put the time on the sheet.

'So then, the second time she called, I gave her advice again. But because there was no time recorded on the first sheet, the solicitor says we have no way of knowing the length of time between the two calls. She said that she could have been in established labour for a long time, and I did nothing about it. I didn't bring her into hospital and she's saying it could be my fault the baby died.'

Will was silent for a minute, digesting everything I had told him.

'What did the hospital say?' he asked, biting his nails.

'A big fat nothing!' I scoffed. 'I wanted to have a talk to one of the managers about it but they're not really interested. They just say it's part of the process, and if I haven't done anything wrong then I've got nothing to worry about.'

It was typical. I hadn't heard a squeak out of the hospital – no briefing or support. Fiona had been off with stress twice already because of the case. Her husband, a corporate lawyer, was gobsmacked that none of us had any training for cases like this. We were just left to sink or swim. We'd never even spoken to the hospital solicitor.

'Now I'm questioning my own actions,' I went on. 'If I had brought her in sooner, would anything have changed? Would there have been a different outcome?'

'But your advice was sound, right?' Will said.

'Yes, I think so.'

'Really, you're fine. Don't worry. That solicitor, she's just trying to rattle you to make you say something stupid. That's what they're paid to do. They think if they back you into a corner, you'll confess or something, but really – how could you be responsible for this baby's death?'

That was the question I kept asking myself over the next few weeks. *Could I be responsible in some way for the baby's death? What if she had been brought in sooner? Would the baby have come out any quicker? Did I miss something? Did I even write it down properly or was there something I left out of my notes?*

The doubts were creeping in and I wondered whether I really was at serious fault. If so, what would the hospital do? *Could I lose my job?* These thoughts kept me awake at night, and in the early hours, all the worst-case scenarios played out in my mind. I would be found guilty of neglect. I'd lose my job. Would I get sent to prison? The significance of that one failure to record something adequately had blown up in my mind to gargantuan proportions.

'Oh, you're always writing!' one husband said to me the week after the call from the solicitor. 'What have you written there? '*Offered a cheese sandwich*'! Seriously? Why do you need to write that down?'

'Trust me, it matters,' I said. 'I've been accused in the past of not feeding people.'

'Ha! Idiots! We wouldn't do that,' he insisted.

I raised one eyebrow. You never know what will happen or how the birth will go – or, subsequently, how a family will react. The UK is a complaining nation these days, so having an accurate and detailed record of what you've said and done is absolutely vital. People simply forget, especially in stressful situations. You just never know when a lapse in memory is going to get you dragged into court!

Fortunately, I was normally too busy to worry about the case while I was on a shift. There was always plenty to do on the ward and, as usual, we were short-staffed. One night, a single mum in labour was brought in by ambulance, along with her five children. We don't usually have a policy about kids in the delivery suite because, after all, if a woman is giving birth at home, then she would have her children with her. Personally, I'm all for letting teenagers into the delivery suite, because if it will put them off having sex and making babies then that makes our job a whole lot easier!

But there's a difference between one or two well-supervised children and five lively unsupervised kids, aged between three and nine, shouting, joking, hitting and pinching each other and generally bringing chaos to a delivery suite.

'This is silly,' Gaby, one of the midwives, complained at the nurses' station. 'We're not bloody babysitters.'

'Well, what is she supposed to do with them?' I countered. 'She can't leave them on their own at home to fend for themselves.'

'I've got an idea,' said Jen. 'Room Twelve is free – it's got a big double bed and a sofa bed. Let's get that set up for them and see if they'll settle down for the night there.'

Gaby was still grumbling about this not being 'her job' as we ushered the children into Room Twelve, put the telly on, fed them sandwiches and fruit, brought some toys down from the children's ward and tried to bed them down for the night.

'It's better this way,' I said to her as we closed the door, reassuring them all we would come and get them when the new baby arrived. 'At least Mum isn't worried about them now and, as long as they're quiet, why shouldn't we look after them? I mean, supporting the mother in labour *is* part of the job.'

* * *

The months dragged on and there was still no resolution to the 'tentorial tear' case. Meanwhile, Fiona had brought in her notice on more than one occasion, saying that she couldn't cope with the stress and simply didn't want to be in the job any more. Somehow, Jen managed to convince her to hang in there, but it wasn't easy. The hospital trust's solicitor called me in to speak to me one morning. I blurted it all out, about failing to put the time on the sheet, and how worried I was about it. I told her my fears and how the solicitor had basically accused me of being responsible for the baby's death. She reassured me that the date and time was not the cause of death, and pointed out that the third phone call Gaynor made to the hospital, when the midwife brought her in, was only a few hours after the first call.

'So, you can see she wasn't left at home in labour for hours,' she concluded. She said that all those involved in the case were on standby to be called to the coroner's court for the hearing, which was due to be held over two days in the middle of March: 14–16 March to be precise.

'But we're going away on the twelfth,' I said. 'That's right slap bang in the middle of our holiday!' Will and I had booked a week in Tenerife with Betty, our first foreign holiday together as a family.

'I'm sorry, Pippa, you'll have to cancel,' she said. 'At the moment, there is a very strong chance you'll be called to give evidence.'

'Strong chance?'

'Well, of course we won't know for certain until nearer the time. Maybe just a day or so in advance.'

I went home to deliver the bad news to Will. He knew that there was nothing I could do about it but he vented nonetheless, furious at the hospital for putting me in this situation with no prior notice. He said he knew how important it was to me but, at this moment, it felt like my job was more important than him, Betty or our life. It was all consuming, and it had begun to affect our family life. Will, who had always been my support, my rock, the person who picked up the pieces when I came home in bits, had finally snapped.

We decided to wait it out and hope that I would be released in the run up to the court date, but twenty-four hours before we were due to fly I still hadn't heard so, reluctantly, we decided to cancel the holiday. There was no question I wouldn't turn up to court. I knew the repercussions would be serious – the judge could put out a warrant out for my arrest and I would lose my job. So that was that. Our first holiday as a family was ruined. We weren't even insured because the court case was classed as a pre-existing issue and not a random event.

Eventually, the day before the case was heard, I was told I didn't actually need to appear – by which time, of course, it was too late, and we'd missed the chance to go away.

Three days after that, the coroner recorded an open verdict. Negligence had not been proven. Relief immediately gave way to anger. All that worrying for nothing! The whole case had put me under a huge amount of unnecessary stress and we'd had to cancel our first foreign holiday in years, all because I'd not written the time on one sheet of paper. It was madness – utter madness. I should have been eliminated from the case from the start, but the fact that the hospital either couldn't or wouldn't defend me made me feel more vulnerable than ever. I was more and more convinced that our hospital trust didn't care about protecting its staff, only its reputation. All of us midwives involved in that case had been left unsupported, without any help from the solicitors representing the hospital. My trust and confidence in the management fell even further during this whole sorry period. If we couldn't rely on the hospital to back us up when we were under attack, perhaps we needed our own advocates.

This, however, would be a cripplingly expensive option. Court cases were becoming more and more common as unhappy families sought resolution to their issues through the courts – and we were in their firing line, without help, training or support. It was like being sent into battle blindfolded and with both hands tied behind our backs. Talk about 'not our job'! I would rather look after an army of unruly children than go through another court case. Meanwhile, the cutbacks increased, leaving us horribly short-staffed at the best of times. We normally had twelve midwives on our unit at any one time, covering the labour ward, postnatal and antenatal wards, but most days we struggled to get eight. It seemed my troubles were far from over.

20

Pressure

Walking out of a side room, where I had just delivered a baby, the LWC, Emily, took me aside and asked me to pop into another as there was a lady about to deliver. My heart sank. I would like to have said no. I really needed to just get on with the two hours' worth of mountainous paperwork I had to complete for the baby I had only just delivered, and continue to provide that lady with care for her first two hours of being a parent.

'Isn't there anyone else?' I asked, but already I could see the hopelessness in her eyes.

'You know I wouldn't ask you if there was, Pippa,' she said, apologetically. 'I know you've just come out of a delivery, but there is literally no one else. I'm sorry.'

'Okay, okay, just give me a minute. Let me get changed, and I want to make sure the breastfeeding support worker comes round to see this lady as soon as she's free.' Usually, I would be the one to help with the first feed but, on this occasion, there was clearly no time. *Would she be okay?*

Would the support worker be free to attend quickly? My mind raced with all the worst-case scenarios as I dived into the staff bathroom to change out of my blood-soaked dress and into a fresh pair of scrubs. My lady needed midwife care at this vital time but there simply were not enough midwives on the ward to give it. This lack of professional attention was becoming a constant struggle and a daily worry to me.

Today we were down to seven midwives due to sickness, stress and general staff shortages. Of these, two midwives were on a full postnatal ward of thirty-two women – and if you're taking the babies into account, the patient total was sixty-four on this one unit alone! Then five midwives were allocated to the labour ward full of labouring women, which was twelve ladies in the rooms and two in pools – all in need of care. On top of that there was the triage to run, which is like our A&E for pregnancy. And we only managed to get up to seven because we called in the two community midwives, which meant our home birth service was currently suspended.

Daytime was always harder on the ward because people wanted to go home. I was constantly being pressured by new parents: *Can I go home? Can I go home now? What am I waiting for?* Every woman on the postnatal ward was always desperate to leave. But I had to explain that our job wasn't just about delivering their baby safely – we had to complete all the necessary checks on the infant before we could discharge them, as well as a lorryload of paperwork. The paediatricians needed to carry out their checks, the hearing screeners had to come, and then there were the physio visits for anyone who had a section or a tear. It can take a while before each of these professionals is able to attend. On a weekend, for example, there's only one paediatrician to cover the maternity ward, A&E, the children's ward, birthing unit and the neonatal unit. That's one paediatrician covering five separate units. Then, if there's an emergency of the kind that could take the one paediatrician off the ward, parents have to wait even longer for their babies to be seen. Most of these checks can be done at home by the community midwife, but if any baby or mother has a suspected infection then a paediatrician must attend before they leave the ward.

The hearing screeners might also have thirty-two women to see, so it takes them time to make their way round everybody, while at the same time the midwives have to carry out maternal checks, baby checks and offer breastfeeding support. I've always loved helping out with breastfeeding wherever I can but, because we were now under so much pressure, that role was falling more and more to the breastfeeding support workers. And in the last two months, we had had to close the unit on no less than three occasions, something our management team weren't happy about because the Trust was fined every time the unit closed. Funnily enough, we never seemed to be short-staffed on management, just midwives . . .

Ten minutes after the first delivery, I had changed and was walking into the other room where a lady called Maggie was about to deliver. Fortunately, I knew her. Maggie was a teaching assistant at Betty's school, and she was also a surrogate mum. This was the second child she was having for the same family. Maggie was lovely – one of those truly special people in the world. She'd already had three of her own children before deciding to give this remarkable gift to another family, and all her births had, thankfully, been without incident.

'Hello, Maggie, how are you getting on?' I grinned, taking a quick scan of her notes. *So far so good.*

'Oh, not too bad,' Maggie puffed. 'Fifth pregnancy! You'd think I'd be used to this by now!'

'She's doing brilliantly,' said Sophie, the 'intended' mother of the new baby. Sophie and Henry were a sweet couple – I'd met them the first time Maggie had acted as their surrogate. They had tried for many years to have a child naturally, as well as going through several rounds of IVF, before discovering that Sophie had a problem with her uterus, which meant she could never carry to term. Four years earlier their fertilised egg had been implanted into Maggie, and that had resulted in the successful birth of their little girl. Now they were expecting a little boy the same way.

Until very recently, our NHS Trust hadn't recognised surrogacy and there were no policy guidelines for midwives. Without any policy in place, we simply had to use our common sense and compassion to guide us. Even now UK law is fairly sparse on the issue. Though it is legal, surrogacy agreements cannot be enforced by law, so if the surrogate changes her mind, there is no legal recourse for the intended parents. The law also states that a surrogate mother retains full parental responsibility of the child until the baby has been legally adopted or there is a parental order in place. Practically, this means the baby must go home with the surrogate mother – we can't allow the 'intended parents' to take the baby without her.

I reviewed Maggie's birth plan – it was fairly straight-forward but lacking in a few details, so I asked her: 'Do you want to hold him first or is the baby going straight to Sophie and Henry?' I recalled the first time we did this: Maggie had the little girl delivered up onto her chest and she then passed the baby to Sophie. At the time she felt it was an important aspect to the surrogacy – she wanted to be the one to 'give' the baby to the new parents. But now Maggie scowled and shook her head.

'No. No, I think he has to go straight to the parents this time,' she said. 'I'm not going to lie, I found it really hard the way we did it last time – holding her and then giving her away. It didn't feel right.'

'Okay,' I said. 'Well, we've set up the room next door for Sophie and Henry so, once the baby is born, we'll take him through to that room and they can have skin-to-skin contact while I stay in here with you and deliver the placenta. Does that work for you, Maggie?'

'Yeah, that's fine,' she said.

I'd already come across several cases of surrogacy – it has become more common in recent years, and we've had a few cases of women carrying children for gay couples. I admire women like Maggie who could put themselves and their bodies through the rigors of pregnancy and birth in order to give the gift of a child to people unable to conceive. Of course, having a baby is easier for some than others, but no matter who you are, it takes a toll on your physical health, and I often wonder about the psychological effects too. Surrogates are not allowed to be paid a fee for their services in this country, only 'reasonable expenses'. We don't ask the amounts involved, but I imagine it is in the thousands in order to make the considerable sacrifice worthwhile.

Once I'd taken Sophie and Henry through to the room next door, I asked Maggie how the pregnancy had been this time round.

'Not bad. This one's a wriggler! Kept me up at night, kicking me under the ribs.'

'Can I ask a question?' I asked tentatively.

'Of course.'

'Is it hard? You know, feeling all the movements, knowing you won't be keeping the baby?'

'No, not really, because I know this baby isn't mine. I know that from the very start, so I have no sense in which I think of the baby as my child. Even so, I'm glad for that separate room. I'm happy to do this – it's an honour, there's no doubt about it – but I'm only human. I think I'd find it difficult to watch them bonding with him just after the birth. I mean, while I'm recovering I'd rather not have to see them together.'

It took just three hours for Maggie to deliver the little boy, and then my student midwife took him straight through to the family while I delivered the placenta. Later, I went to see Sophie and Henry and their happiness was contagious. I could see why Maggie chose to do this. She had made their dreams come true – after so much heartache and disappointment, here were two beautiful children, the family they had always yearned for. These were two of the most wanted children I have ever met. Just twenty-four hours later they would all leave the hospital together, as our protocols prevented Sophie and Henry from taking the little boy without Maggie, his legal guardian. But for now, I had another two hours of paperwork ahead of me, meaning I would be home late – again! By the time

Pressure

I eventually managed to crawl home, my head was fuzzy from dehydration and I hadn't eaten properly in hours, but the first thing I did as always when I got into the house was head straight to the loo.

Bloody hell – I can't seem to get off. It's like a waterfall! Suddenly it hit me that I hadn't peed in sixteen hours. I hadn't had a chance. Betty now bowled into the bathroom.

'Mummy! Mummy! Mummy!' she yelled excitedly.

'Oh, just give me a minute!' I snapped, as she tried to put her arms around my knees for a cuddle. I pushed her away.

'Hey!' Will admonished. 'She's just pleased to see you, that's all. She hasn't seen you all day.'

'I'm on the toilet here, in case you hadn't noticed!' I retorted. But then I saw Betty's crestfallen little face and instantly regretted my outburst. She was only six, after all. She didn't understand.

'Oh, sweetheart, I'm sorry.' *Why am I so snappy? This isn't like me.* I fell into bed, exhausted and desperate for rest. But sleep, like on most nights, again eluded me. My eyes remained stubbornly open as my mind replayed all the events of the day: *did I do everything right? Did I make the right notes? Were my ladies getting the right aftercare?*

Everything felt so disjointed these days, it was impossible to see a woman through from the birth to being discharged and ensure she'd had all the checks, care and help. I felt like one of those circus plate-spinners with a dozen plates spinning on poles. You know that it's only a question of taking your eye off one of those poles for a second and then – disaster! The digital clock on my bedside table clicked slowly through the early morning hours: 3.15 a.m., 4.22 a.m, 5.19 a.m. At some point, I dropped off and managed a couple

253

of hours sleep, but the next morning, when Betty bounded into our bedroom, I felt groggy and unwell, hungover almost.

'Oh God, I feel like hell warmed up,' I groaned to Will. I'd been fighting off a cold for a couple of weeks now, but my nose was completely blocked and my throat sore.

'You don't look great,' he confirmed.

"I didn't sleep well either and now, *urgh*, I'm full of cold.'

'Why don't you take the day off sick?'

'Don't be silly.'

'No, seriously,' he insisted.

'You know the answer to that, Will. If I take one more day off sick before January then I'll be put on Stage Two.'

There was a strict sickness protocol at our hospital trust. If you took up to two days off sick within six months you were officially on Stage 1 of the protocol. Any more than that and it automatically tipped you onto Stage 2 – then you were called in for a 'capability meeting' with your line manager and HR, to assess whether you were actually capable of working any more. In other words, if you were properly sick then your job was at risk. It meant we were all terrified of taking sick days. I had already had two days off in August for a nasty chest infection, so now I was on Stage 1. If I went off sick now, I was worried I could lose my job. I toyed with the idea of taking a day of Emergency Annual Leave to recover, but realised we were already horrendously short-staffed this week, and if I went off at short notice, it would be a nightmare for the rest of the team. So, I dragged myself out of bed, threw down a cup of Day Nurse, pulled on my uniform and drove to work.

Halfway through the morning, I was on all fours delivering a baby, my nose streaming, when I asked my student midwife to assist. Very quietly I whispered to her: 'Alison, will you please wipe my nose? I don't want this baby to be covered in snot the moment she arrives in this world!'

Alison dashed off to the bathroom for some toilet paper, came back and actually wiped my nose to save this baby entering this world covered in my phlegm! Afterwards, I slumped in the staffroom, feeling completely wrecked. I just hoped there wouldn't be any major complications today as I was already on my knees.

'You don't look full of beans today,' Helen remarked, as she noticed me hunched over in a corner.

'Sick,' I rasped.

'Go home then.'

'No, I can't. I took two days off last month. One more day and I'll be on Stage Two.'

When I got to the end of my shift, I felt utterly drained, my eyes were streaming, nose blocked. The strict sickness protocol, whilst set up to stop people from taking *unnecessary* days off, was also preventing people taking very *necessary* days off, too. We're human, after all, and we're working in an environment where sickness, bugs and infections are rife – it's only natural that we will occasionally fall ill. And being punished for that contributes to the 'stress epidemic' that is engulfing our hospital wards. I am absolutely certain that there would be less staff suffering from stress and depression if they weren't so worried about us taking one or two days off sick for genuine reasons. If the NHS accepts that its staff will sometimes go sick, then perhaps they will actually hold onto them for longer.

Of course, Helen understood. We both knew midwives and nurses who had been 'let go' after capability meetings.

'Yes, and I've got to be honest, I really don't want to lose you today,' she mused. 'Did you hear about the overdose?'

'No. What happened?'

'Drug error. Two midwives, just qualified, were doing the drug rounds last night and there was nobody senior around, as the LWC had to step in to manage a delivery. They were due to administer meds to a baby born with a suspected infection, and instead of giving the zero point five mil dose, they gave baby a five mil dose.'

'Oh no!'

'Yes. Thankfully, I checked their notes during handover and spotted the error, and the baby went straight to neonatal. I think she's fine – no damage done – but both of the midwives are really shaken up.'

'God, that could have been serious.'

'It *was* serious, but that's what happens when we're understaffed, there's no senior team to give oversight and newly qualified midwives are left in charge. I feel sorry for them. It's not their fault, but I don't doubt they'll be hauled in by the Navy Blues for a dressing down.'

Helen was right – without enough senior staff around, mistakes were becoming a more frequent occurrence. Quite often on the labour ward we call for a second midwife when the lady is going to deliver, just in case we need a second pair of hands if, for example, the baby needs resuscitation. But recently I'd pulled my buzzer and nobody had turned up. Most of the time, that's fine, and you can deliver the baby on your own without any problems. But you never know what's going to happen. That's the point about labour, it's unpredictable, and it's reassuring to have an extra pair of hands, just in case. In the past we had been stopped from making up the numbers by calling in agency staff, because they were so expensive, but in the last few months that rule had been abandoned. We were now calling in agency staff all the time because we simply didn't have the numbers to run the ward. It made a difference but, even so, there were times when it would simply be better to have our own midwives, because there were certain procedures that agency staff weren't allowed to carry out, like checking drugs, giving intravenous infusions and epidural top-ups. And on one occasion, an agency healthcare assistant had actually put a lady's health in jeopardy.

It had happened after a fairly straightforward delivery. The baby was on the mother's chest and I was just delivering the placenta when she started bleeding. Blood gushed out of her, pouring down the bottom of the bed, quickly forming a large puddle on the floor. It was instantaneous; she lost a good litre in seconds, so I put my hand on her tummy straight away. That amount usually means it's uterine. Inside the body, after a birth, the uterus is a big open-wound site, and the body's way of stopping that bleeding is for the uterus to contract and compress it. But sometimes, if the body has worked too hard in labour, it just doesn't do that – it becomes relaxed and fails to contract. So, we do compressions, pressing on the woman's tummy in an attempt to keep the uterus contracted and stop the bleeding. I pulled the emergency buzzer. Now, normally when you pull the emergency buzzer the whole team piles in – at least ten members of staff. But on this occasion we had an agency healthcare support worker, who had been into the room earlier on, during the delivery. She was one of the first in the room with another midwife, and asked me, 'What's happened?'

'She's bleeding!' I replied.

And for some reason I still don't understand to this day, the healthcare worker failed to appreciate the seriousness of the situation and simply turned on her heels, walked back out again, and announced to the rest of the team behind her: 'No emergency here. It's a false alarm.'

I heard her say those words and it was like everything suddenly went into slow motion. I recall the panic in the eyes of the other midwife who had come in with the healthcare assistant. I shook my head at her, and she immediately turned around and ran out after the healthcare assistant.

'NO. NO. NO! It's not a false alarm. Come back. Come back! We have a lady bleeding. Get back here!'

She had to round them all up again to get them back in the room, but thank God she was there, because, if she hadn't done that, we could have been in serious trouble. When it comes to bleeding, every second counts.

Then the registrar rushed in, pulled on a pair of gloves and started bimanual compressions. This is where they put a fist in the uterus and the other on top of the tummy in order to manually compress it from both sides to stem the bleeding until we can get some drugs into her to help the uterus contract.

'Forty units of oxytocin!' he shouted out. Then: 'Eight hundred milligrams of misoprostol!'

And we all got to work, administering three different types of drugs to stop the bleeding and contract the uterus. It took some time but eventually the bleeding did stop, but not before she had lost a good two litres. It doesn't sound a lot but it *looks* a lot and is an alarming sight. I've seen big blood losses, sixteen litres in theatre, but there, it's all being sucked away, or we do self-salvage (that's where we hoover up the blood, filter it, put it in a bag and then give it back to the woman). Two litres is a frightening amount of blood loss when it's pooling on the floor.

* * *

I somehow got through the day without any other major incident, but I had so many women to look after, so much to think about, that I left that day with a horrible headache. Too much to think about. Too many plates in the air. How could I possibly give all these women the care they needed when I was stretched so thin? It would make a difference if a Band 8 helped out occasionally. A drug round takes forty-five minutes and we have to do three every day shift, so even if a Band 8 just stepped in to do the drug rounds, it would free us up massively to look after our ladies properly.

Once again, I drove home in a fog, my mind so overstretched and fractured that I had nothing left in the tank for Betty or Will.

'I'm going to bed,' I grunted at Will as soon as I fell in the front door.

'But I've made supper . . .' Will cried out as I trudged up the stairs.

'I'll have it later. Sorry . . . need to sleep.'

'Mummy!' Betty called out.

'Not now, Betty . . . not now . . .'

21

The Sound of
Falling Plates

What's wrong with me? My heart raced, my stomach was in knots and I could barely catch my breath. I was pinned to my seat, unable to move, unable to get out of the car. *Shit. What's happening?*

It was a chilly, misty morning in early November 2018, and I'd driven to work as usual for the 7 a.m. handover, but the moment I switched off my engine in the hospital car park, I could feel panic rising in my chest. I willed myself to turn the handle of the door and get out, but I couldn't. I just couldn't move. My breathing came in short, shallow bursts. I was paralysed. *I can't do it. I just can't do this any more.* I looked over to the maternity unit where I was due to spend another twelve hours and all I could feel was overwhelming fear. I didn't know what to do – it was the first time I had ever felt like this. Shakily, I pulled my mobile phone out of my bag and dialled my mum's number.

'Hello, love – are you alright?' Her familiar voice offered a touch of reassurance.

'Mum, I'm in the car park at work and I just . . . I don't want to go in.'

'Why? What do you mean?'

'I feel like I'm going to do something wrong. I feel like I'm an accident waiting to happen.'

'Ah, love, you've been working too hard. So *don't* go in. Take a day off sick. Just look after yourself, Pippa. You need a break.'

'I can't take a day off, Mum. I'm already on Stage 1. If I take another day off before January, I'll be sent for a capability meeting.'

'Then take a deep breath and just focus on getting the work done. You'll be alright. You're just having a moment. Come on – deep breath. You're fine, love. Honestly. You're fine.'

I closed my eyes and took a deep breath in. Mum was right. I was just having a moment. I'd be alright in a minute. We hung up and I took a couple more deep breaths until the panic had passed. I managed to get out the car and walk to the unit. *Just focus on the work,* I kept telling myself. And that's what I tried to do.

But from the moment I arrived on the ward, the workload was overwhelming. I wanted to do a good job, to ensure that every woman I looked after got the proper care she needed, but since we were short-staffed again, that was impossible. Leaving one room where a woman had just delivered to go into another room for a delivery meant my mind was constantly divided. *What happens to the other lady? Is she going to be alright when I'm with this other one? Who's to say she's not going to haemorrhage while I'm delivering this other baby? Has she had something to eat or drink? Has she had some support for the breastfeeding? Plates in the air, plates in the air – all spinning, spinning, spinning. Surely, it can't go on like this . . .* And still the work piled up.

'Pippa, can you just see this lady?'

'Pippa, can you have a look at room number twelve?'

'Pippa, can you do the drugs round?'

Normally, I would find a way to accommodate all the requests of the senior team, but today was not a good day.

'FOR HEAVEN'S SAKE, CAN'T YOU SEE I'VE GOT MY HANDS FULL!' I snapped at Laura, when she approached me the third time that morning.

'You know I wouldn't normally ask . . .' she stuttered.

'No, you *would* ask. You *do* ask all time. I've already got three ladies I'm looking after. Ask someone else!'

And then I stomped off down the corridor to attend to one of the women who was about to get in the pool. Once I was in the room with the family, I was all smiles, of course. We're very good at that, us midwives, making it seem like everything is fine, even if there is an impending disaster on the horizon. Nobody would have guessed there was anything wrong at all. I smiled, laughed and joked with family, carried out all my checks and observations and answered all their questions. But underneath I was seething: *How dare she! Why does she think she can dump everything on me? It's the same every day. She knows I've already got three ladies – it's unfair to ask me to do more!*

Two hours later, I was rooted to the spot in the corridor, holding a bunch of towels, wondering who they were for and which room I was meant to be in. I couldn't think straight. *Come on, Pippa. Come on. Get it together.* But my thoughts were all jumbled up, and for some reason the answer refused to come. *I've got these towels – but who are they for?* I must have been standing there, scowling at the floor for ages, before I felt a soft hand on my shoulder.

'Pippa? Are you okay, Pippa?' Helen asked gently. It was the straw that broke the camel's back. I burst into floods of tears.

'I can't do it any more,' I sobbed. 'I just . . . I can't cope. It's too much.'

Helen steered me out of the corridor and into the staffroom where she sat me down on the sofa and handed me tissues as I cried and cried. It was like a dam had burst inside me.

'Pippa, this is not like you,' she said. 'You need to see the doctor, straight away.'

She was right. I had never snapped at a colleague like I'd done earlier. I was always a happy, smiley person. No matter how pressed I was, I was never normally rude to anyone. I wasn't coping and I couldn't hide it any more. The chronic staff shortages, the overwork, the constant stress of targets and compliance, not getting my breaks, the sleepless nights, never finishing on time, having so much on my plate, it had all built up.

The buzzer went and my heart sank.

'It's one of my ladies,' I sighed. 'I have to . . .'

'No, don't move,' Helen insisted. 'I'll go. You call your GP now and make an appointment. You can't go on like this.' I sank back down into the sofa, grateful for her help.

'Are you sure?' I asked.

'Yes, make that appointment now.'

I did as Helen instructed: I called my GP and managed to get an appointment to see her the next morning at

The Sound of Falling Plates

9 a.m. Just knowing that I had the appointment gave me the strength to get through the rest of the day and, somehow, I stumbled through the afternoon, desperately trying to hold it together, even though my head felt it was about to explode most of the time. At the end of my shift, I approached the LWC.

'I'm really sorry, Laura, for losing my temper earlier,' I said. 'I'm not feeling myself at the moment. I've not been sleeping well and, I don't know, it just got too much.'

'It's okay, Pippa, I understand. We're all feeling it at the moment. It doesn't help that we're chronically understaffed. I just wish we had one day, *one day*, where we had enough midwives on.'

'I know, I know.'

'It's getting beyond a joke.'

A joke? I thought about that as I left the ward, got in my car and headed home. *A joke?* I couldn't remember the last time I had laughed – a proper belly laugh. I couldn't remember the last time I had found anything remotely funny.

At 9 a.m. the next day, I looked up at the clock in the doctor's surgery. It was exactly the same type as we had on our wards – *tick, tick, tick tick*. I watched the red second-hand moving round the clock face and, without warning, my eyes began to well up. Sitting there, in the GP's office, I finally felt able to be honest about what was going on in my head.

'At work, I just feel that there's so much going on,' I explained. 'I'm afraid it's only a matter of time before I make a mistake. It's bound to happen. I can feel it. You can't take on that much work at once and keep on top of it all the time; it's just not possible. So then I'll do something wrong and maybe a lady will bleed out or something will go wrong with the baby and who'll get the blame? Not the doctors, not the consultants. It will be me! If one of us makes the tiniest mistake, it's never the consultant's fault or the fact that we don't have enough support from the senior team. It's the midwives who get called in for the capability meetings, who get suspended, who go to court. I've seen it! I see it all the time.

'They put you through this. You go to coroner's court, and you're under all this pressure for no reward. You're not trained to deal with it. There are no classes for what to say in court or how to conduct yourself. It's like . . . one minute you're doing your job, and the next you're jumping into a pool of the unknown, and all the stress of dealing with it is unbelievable. And if you say the wrong thing or the wrong *word* even, it comes back to bite you on the arse because you've got managers on managers who will filter it down and make your life hell. Then where are you? Your whole career ruined, flushed down the toilet because of a wrong word and it's impossible sometimes. You don't know what to do and that's how I feel now . . . I just don't know what to do. I don't go to work to do a bad job. I go to work to give it my all and give the women what they deserve. But I can't do that right now.

'And my brain doesn't feel right. I can't smile. I can't be happy. I want to feel happy with Betty, but I can't. I'm just so exhausted all the time, but at the same time I don't sleep because my mind is always racing and I'm going back over the day and thinking, *have I done the right thing?* Or, *did I write the paperwork correctly?* And it just plays on my mind all night long. I get home and I'm forever messaging colleagues or ringing work in the middle of the night to see how the ladies I looked after are doing if I wasn't there for the delivery.'

I didn't even know what I was even saying any more – I was just babbling. Suddenly I stopped. The doctor looked at me, her brows furrowed with concern.

'It sounds very much like you are suffering from stress and depression, Pippa,' she said seriously. 'You need rest, and you need to be away from the environment which is causing all this. I can sign you off work today.'

'Sign me off work?' I repeated slowly. *Am I depressed?* It never occurred to me that I could be depressed. It seemed so unlikely. This is not *me*. I had an idea of myself as a happy person and this didn't seem to fit. Suddenly my head was swimming. *If she signs me off work that will only make the staff shortage problem even worse for those left behind. How can I just abandon my colleagues? Surely this will put even more pressure on the staff.* I was flooded with guilt.

'But we can't afford to lose another midwife,' I objected.

'That is not your problem, Pippa. You are not responsible for what is happening at the hospital. You are only responsible for yourself, and right now you have to focus on getting well again.'

It was true. I felt like I was failing at everything right now. I was a shit midwife, a shit mother and a shit partner to Will. I hadn't even been out with any friends recently because I just felt rotten all the time. *Fine. If she says I'm depressed, then maybe she's right. I've got to do something because I can't go on like this.* All the fight had left me.

'Okay . . . what do I do?'

'I'm signing you off sick for a month. Please take this note

267

to your managers. And I'm also writing out a prescription for a course of antidepressants. I have started you on a low dose. This is not a miracle cure, but I want to see you back in two weeks to see how you're coping. Go home, Pippa. Go home and rest.'

* * *

Is this what depression feels like? I don't know. All I know is that I can't move. I feel utterly drained of energy and all the things I used to do or get pleasure from have stopped. I pulled the duvet tighter around me and turned on my side, away from the sunlight streaming through the blinds. It was around midday, I wasn't exactly sure, and I'd been in bed since taking Betty to school at 8.30 am this morning. Even that felt like a huge effort. Just getting her up, making her breakfast and getting her dressed and ready for school was enough to sap the last remaining energy from me. I dragged myself to the school gates, kissed her goodbye and then hauled myself back home to bed. It had been two weeks since the appointment with the GP and from that point it seemed I had gone into a full-scale collapse. At first, I was unsure about taking the antidepressants. Was it really necessary, I wondered? But Will said I should trust the doctor so, as soon as I picked up the prescription, I started on the medication.

Downstairs, I was aware of the overflowing washing basket, the dishes piling up next to the sink and the toys scattered across the living room floor, but I had no motivation to do anything about any of it. From the pit of my stomach to the tips of my fingers, I felt rotten, utterly rotten. And my inability to do normal, everyday tasks made me feel guilty too, compounding those feelings of helplessness and inadequacy. I had snapped at Betty last night, and Will, too – of course, I immediately apologised, but I felt like I was no longer in control of my emotions. I was always apologising these days! Now Will had gone to work, Betty was in school, and I lay in bed, unable to get enough energy to get up and walk the dog.

An hour later, I dragged myself to the toilet then went straight back to bed. I texted Mum: *Having a bad day. Please pick up Betty from school later.* She replied straight away: *Sure – wish you better, darling.* Her message brought on a fresh bout of tears. Then I switched on my laptop and went onto my Netflix account. I was halfway through the fourth series of *Breaking Bad*. It was about all I could manage at that moment – lying in bed, binge-watching TV. Later, I would move onto *Better Call Saul*. I watched so many American dramas during those bleak times, but to this day I can't remember a thing about the plotlines or characters – my brain couldn't retain the information from one day to the next. Later, Will came in from work after collecting Betty from my mum's, made us all tea then put our daughter to bed. Before she had her night-time story, she crept in to see me, and when she saw my eyes open, she threw herself on top of me.

'Hope you feel better tomorrow, Mummy,' she whispered in my ear. 'Then we can play.'

It broke my heart.

'I'm sorry,' I wept to Will later that evening,

'Shhh . . . it's okay,' he soothed. 'It's not your fault.'

'I feel like I'm letting everyone down.'

'You're not, you're really not. You're not well, love. That's what the doctor says, and I can see it myself. You're not yourself. Don't worry. We'll get through this together. We're a team, right?'

I smiled weakly at him.

'I don't know what I'd do without you.'

'Come 'ere,' he said, as he pulled me into a gigantic bear hug.

But in the early hours of the morning, I found myself wide awake, staring at the moon, wondering what had happened to me. I used to be a happy person, so full of joy, loving my life, loving my job. I didn't recognise myself any more. *How long will this go on? How long before I'm better?*

Though I'd started the antidepressants immediately, the doctor had warned me that it would take at least four weeks before they would start to work. She had also put my name down for cognitive behavioural therapy (CBT), but there was currently a three-month waiting list to see a therapist, which meant I had no hope of getting therapy in the immediate future. Meanwhile, the depression left me catatonic most days. So, a month after I went off sick, the doctor signed me off for a further six weeks. It took everything I had to go into work to hand them the sick note. I still felt so drained of energy and, on top of that, being in the hospital made me feel horrendously guilty because I knew how much pressure everyone was under. I had put on weight too. Lying in bed for a month, watching box sets and eating takeaways because I had no energy to cook had meant the pounds had piled on, so I felt embarrassed and self-conscious of my appearance. But I had no choice – after the first month off work, I was instructed to attend a 'keep in touch' meeting with my manager.

When I arrived in Lina's office that morning, she gave

me a massive grin and exclaimed: 'Wow! You look so much better, Pippa. Are you feeling better now?'

'No, not really,' I mumbled. *Christ, and now I feel bad for not feeling better!*

'Oh, I'm sorry to hear that,' she replied, smiling insincerely.

'I've got a letter from my GP to give you. She's signing me off work for another six weeks.'

'Right.' The smile fled from her face as she took the envelope.

'She's upping my antidepressants.'

'Okay, well, we hope that helps. In the meantime, it might help for you to pay a visit to our Occupational Health Department. We have a resilience programme in place, and it has certainly been beneficial to others with similar issues.'

'Yes, I will,' I agreed. I was willing to try anything – in truth, I was desperate for help. More than anything I wanted to be back to my normal self, back to the old Pippa from before.

'Okay, well, if there's nothing else?' she said brightly, and with that she turned back to her work. Conversation over, a sign that it was time for me to go. I scurried out, desperate to leave the unit without being seen. I hadn't yet told any of my friends and colleagues what was happening. I left their kind messages and texts unanswered. The truth was, I was ashamed and embarrassed about being ill. I didn't want to be the talk of the unit, so I raced out and went straight home. Back to bed.

As Christmas approached, I realised I couldn't face going shopping for presents. The only time I left the house these days was to walk Betty to school and back, and even that took it out of me. As well as fighting the constant fatigue, I was frightened of telling people I knew that I was off work with depression. I'd told my immediate family, of course, and they were incredibly supportive. Both my parents, and Will's, offered to take Betty after school and at the weekends while I struggled with the most basic tasks. But I couldn't face telling anyone else. Just the thought of going to Asda and bumping into people I knew sent my heart racing. The idea of Christmas shopping brought on a dizzying panic attack. So, I ordered Betty's presents online and wrapped them from my bed.

At least I can cook a decent Christmas dinner, I told myself in the run up to the big day. *At least I can do that for my daughter.* We had decided it would just be the three of us this year, as I had no stomach for a large family get-together, but I was keen that at least we would share a nice turkey dinner with all the trimmings. But it seemed the harder I tried, the worse everything got. I'd prepped all the vegetables the night before and had even made pigs in blankets, Betty's favourite, and my own homemade stuffing. But on the day itself, we had several power cuts and the oven kept going off, which meant we couldn't get the food cooked.

'Oh, for heaven's sake!' I exploded after yet another power cut left us in near total darkness. 'Why is everything so hard? It's just a posh Sunday dinner and I can't even get that right.'

'Hey, stop beating yourself up!' Will objected. 'It's a power cut. These things happen. It's not personal.'

'I just wanted one nice day together,' I wept.

'We *are* having a nice day together,' Will insisted. 'Betty loves her presents. She's having a lovely time. Relax! We're not going to starve.'

The Sound of Falling Plates

Luckily, Betty didn't witness my outburst in the kitchen, and after we finally got the dinner on the table, I took myself upstairs for a long bath. There, in the solitude of the bathroom, I let out the tears that had threatened to overwhelm me during the day. Afterwards, I wrapped myself in a dressing gown and collapsed onto the bed, where I fell immediately asleep. Will woke me at 8 p.m. with a cup of tea and a slice of Christmas cake.

'Betty wants a kiss goodnight,' he said gently, so I went into her room to tuck her in and kiss her goodnight. She was lying in bed, clutching the brand-new cuddly unicorn she had got from Father Christmas.

'Did Santa get you everything you wanted this year?' I asked her.

'Mmm-hmm,' she answered, nodding. 'Did he get you what you wanted, Mummy?'

'Yeah, course he did,' I said, and swallowed hard.

'I don't think the pills are working,' I confided to Will later that night. 'I don't feel any different. I feel just as bad as before.'

'You're still not yourself,' he agreed. 'Maybe we need to go back to the doctors and see what they say.'

22

Slow Progress

It was January 2019, the start of the New Year, and I wanted to tell my family that I was well again, that I was back at work with renewed vigour, getting high on that unbeatable excitement of delivering new babies into the world. I wanted to tell them that I had recovered and that my ill health was just a small bump in the road. But I couldn't. I had been off sick for two months now and I wasn't ready to go back. The doctor had upped my dosage of antidepressants, but the pills gave me headaches and made me feel sick. Will encouraged me to do something for myself once a week, but it was almost like I had forgotten what I liked to do. For so long, all I had done was go to work, come home and look after Betty. What were my interests? I didn't seem to have any. I didn't fancy socialising, I couldn't face going to the gym, so I started swimming at the local pool on 'ladies' night'. It was the only way I could bear to get into a swimming costume.

Midway through January, I attended the Resilience Training session held by the Occupational Health

Department in the hospital. By now, I was desperate for help, so as soon as I sat down in the small office of a pleasant-looking young woman wearing the name badge *Caroline*, I spilled out all my worries.

'I hate this,' I said. 'I hate being off work. I've been doing this job over half my life, since I was seventeen. It's all I've ever known. I love it. I love everything about it, and because I've been doing it a long time now, I know that I have the skills and the experience to do it well. So I do consider myself a good midwife, but I have seen *plenty* of good midwives go through hell and end up in court because they've been put under such pressure they've made mistakes, or something has gone wrong and the blame has been put on them, even when it is not their fault. The thing is – when we're short-staffed all the time then mistakes are bound to happen. And it's frightening. To be really honest with you, it means when I go into work I'm constantly on edge. I'm constantly worried. Is that right? Is it right that I can't focus properly on my job and give the lady I'm delivering the right care because I'm worried all the time?'

Caroline listened patiently as I confided my darkest fears, nodding and making the occasional note in her pad. Then, once I'd talked myself to a standstill, she put on a very *serious* face and said: 'Philippa, we understand you are struggling with the workload, and that is why we've developed this training programme in order to help you cope better. Now, if you'd just like to turn this way . . .' She stood up and crossed to the back of the room where there was a wall-mounted computer screen. She dimmed the lights and clicked a handheld device and a colourful slide appeared on the screen behind her: 'STRESS: RECOGNISING THE SIGNS', read the title.

Slow Progress

'Now, the first thing we need to learn when dealing with a stressful situation is how to recognise the signs of stress,' she started. She was actually reading the words directly off the slide! And for the next hour, Caroline talked me through her PowerPoint presentation of 'How to Cope with Stress', helpfully listing all the different ways of tackling stress, including breathing exercises, taking regular breaks, staying positive and speaking to the senior team leaders. We went from that to 'Strategies for a Stress-free Life', and here Caroline's recommendations ranged from changing my diet to cutting back on alcohol, drinking more water, taking up yoga and meditation and 'talking things through with a friend'. I found I really didn't have to bother reading the slides at all as, rather helpfully, Caroline read them out, word for word.

I was dumbfounded. At one point, I even span around in my chair, checking the room for hidden cameras: *was this some sort of stupid prank?* Christ, I could get this rubbish from the pages of any woman's magazine! Drink more water? Take up yoga? What a joke! I couldn't believe I'd left the house for this. Sitting there, listening to her reel off a pre-prepared list, I felt patronised and utterly humiliated. After all, I'd poured out my soul to this woman and her response was to read out a scripted presentation. The worst thing was it was all so unfair. I mean, why put all the emphasis on me and what I should be doing? Why all the emphasis on the individual to fix the situation? Where were the stress-busting strategies that the hospital could act on like, say, oh, I don't know: employing more midwives?

The presentation went on for an hour and a half, and after she finished up, she turned the lights back up and asked if I had any questions. I just shook my head. What could she tell me? She wasn't a qualified therapist in any way – I didn't know what she was but she certainly didn't appear to be medically trained. She was just there to recite a presentation, parrot-style, which had probably been written by someone else.

'Okay, well, you've done the training now, so you should be alright to go back to work,' she concluded.

What? Is she for real?

For a second, I was too taken aback to speak. Then it hit me. I had got the wrong idea of what this was all about. I had come here thinking that 'resilience training' was going to be therapy for me. I thought it was about trying to help *me*. It wasn't. It was about helping *the hospital* by putting me back to work.

'It's all very well you *saying* that I'm ready to go back to work, Caroline, but you don't know what's going on in my head,' I said slowly. 'You don't know anything about me. You've just talked at me for ninety minutes. But I'm watching your PowerPoint like I watch programmes on Netflix. It's going in one ear and out the other. You haven't done anything to help me. My doctor says I'm not well and I'll take her advice, thanks, not yours. I'll come back when I feel ready, not when you say so.'

'Okay, that's fine,' she said sweetly. 'But I do have to make recommendations to your manager.'

'On what basis, exactly?'

'On the basis that you have completed the training. So I am recommending a phased return within one or two weeks.'

Oh, for fuck's sake!

I got up to leave. 'You recommend whatever you like,

Slow Progress

Caroline. I'll return to work when a qualified professional tells me I'm ready. Not on the basis of . . . whatever this is!'

Two weeks later, I was called back into work for a 'review' with Lina. Yet again, I had to face the uncomfortable sight of watching my colleagues run around like lunatics as the staff shortages continued as, once more, I came armed with another sick note from my doctor, who had increased my dosage of antidepressants for a second time.

'And how are you feeling today, Pippa?' she asked. 'I understand you've completed the Resilience Training. So, are you ready for work?'

'No.'

'Well, shall we say you'll come back in two weeks then?'

'No. The doctor says I'm still depressed and has signed me off for another six weeks.' I handed her the letter, which seemed to prompt a chilling effect in the room.

'I see,' she said, reading the note.

'I'll come back when I'm ready,' I went on. 'And you know what – I'm off work for a reason and you keep bringing me back in! I come in here, I see that this place is understaffed and everyone's struggling, and it makes me feel bad. And that puts me under even more pressure than before. I've spoken to my union rep and she says there's no reason I should be made to come in for these reviews. If you need to communicate with me, please do it on email, and when I'm ready to come back, trust me, you'll be the first to know.'

* * *

The truth was, I didn't know if I was ever coming back. Midwifery had been my life up until now, but every time I walked back onto the ward I felt sick to my stomach. Could I carry on doing the job if it made me ill? Will's income could probably cover us for a little while, but he was freelance, and we couldn't rely on him bringing in a regular salary. We had to meet the mortgage somehow – so I started to consider other jobs. I looked into teaching positions, nursing and various other roles that might suit my skill-set, as I struggled through another couple of difficult weeks. I didn't want to talk about how I felt any more – frankly, I was sick of hearing myself complain of how sick I felt. Then, one morning in February, Will made a suggestion.

'Why don't you write it down? If you're feeling like shit, and you don't want to talk about it, why don't you write down what you're feeling?'

'Write what?' I asked.

'Whatever you like! Whatever's bothering you, whatever's in your head. Just get it out. You never know, it could help.'

When Will had left for the day, I thought about what he'd said. I'd never enjoyed writing before. In fact, I had struggled to complete the academic side of my midwifery course (essays brought me out in a cold sweat) but this was different. I wouldn't be writing essays. As Will suggested, I could just write whatever was in my head. So, I picked up an old lined notepad, made myself a cup of tea, sat down at my desk and started to write: 'My name is Philippa George and I'm a midwife, except today I'm not . . .'

Four hours later the phone rang, and, to my surprise, I found I had covered twelve sheets of paper.

'Oh my God!' I said, when I picked up the phone to Will. He regularly called throughout the day to check on me. 'I've been writing this whole time, ever since you left.'

'Really?'

'Yes, I did what you suggested. I just started writing and then I found I couldn't stop!'

'What did you write?'

'Oh, loads of things! Loads of stuff about the babies I've delivered, and the people I've met, and all the good things, Will. I've really enjoyed it.'

'It sounds like it. You sound different. Your voice . . . you sound really upbeat.'

'Yeah, yeah I know.'

The next day, I picked up my pen and wrote again. I wrote about training with Bev, about my friends, and the way we helped each other on the ward. I wrote about the surprise babies, the tragedies, the good times, about Sam, Helen, Jen, Angela, Lina; my anger and sadness, the court cases, the workload, the mistakes and my myriad of experiences. It all came pouring out of me and, by the end of the day, I was drained but I felt better than I had in ages. The next day I wrote again. And the day after that . . . and slowly, gradually, something seemed to lift. Maybe it was the writing, maybe it was the antidepressants finally kicking in, but it felt like I could see the sunshine again. When I walked outside, I could feel its warmth on my skin. When Betty did something funny, I laughed – a real laugh. A big genuine belly laugh. And I knew that something, *something* was changing for the better.

* * *

A week later, I forced myself to do the weekly shop at Asda. It was a big deal and no big deal at the same time. Of course, everyone does a supermarket shop once a week – it's normal. Only I hadn't been out in the world for months, and it took all of my courage just to do that very normal, ordinary thing.

That's the weird thing about mental illness – it can isolate you, make you feel even more like an alien because it robs you of your ability to do the things everyone else takes for granted. It took so much effort just to get out of the car and force myself to walk round the aisles without succumbing to panic.

Since I live in a smallish town, it was almost inevitable that I would bump into someone I knew, so, when it happened, I was relieved to find it was Sarah, an old friend I'd lost touch with in recent months. She seemed very pleased to see me, and when she asked how I'd been, I felt strong enough to tell the truth.

'I've not been great, you know, Sarah. Actually, I've been off work the last few months with stress.'

'Oh God, Pippa, I'm really sorry.'

'Yeah, thanks. It's been a bit of a hard time.'

'I'd like to see you so we can catch up properly. How about we arrange to go out sometime?'

I took a deep breath: 'Yeah, I'd like that. Send me a text and we'll sort something out.'

It was the first time I had talked to anyone outside my immediate family about what I'd been going through – and it wasn't as bad as I'd feared. In fact, just seeing Sarah again made me realise how much I'd missed my mates. Three days later, Sarah and I went out for a drink. I told her everything and she caught me up on her life too. I came back feeling loads better. A week after that, she and two other friends from school dragged me to a '70s night at the local club. I felt a bit shy and self-conscious to begin with, but after a couple of drinks, I let go my inhibitions and had a really good boogie on the dance floor. It was just what I needed!

Slow Progress

All throughout February, and most of March, I felt myself getting better bit by bit. I wrote most days, and in the afternoons I took the dog for a walk.

'Can I read this?' Will asked one day. He had my writing book in his hand. For a moment I hesitated. *Was there anything in there I didn't want him to see? Did I have any dark secrets from my past he didn't know about?* I thought for a second before replying: 'Sure. I don't think it's any good. It just helps to get it out. And you know, thinking back about all the good stuff is nice too. It's been like taking a trip down memory lane.'

'I'd like to see it anyway.'

'Be my guest.'

Two hours later, Will came to find me while I was watching TV.

'This is really good,' he said. 'I can see why you like doing your job. Loads of drama!'

'Yeah, it's amazing really. I think that's why the writing has been so good for me. It's reminded me why I love being a midwife.'

'So, you think you'll be going back?'

'Yeah, I think I should give it a go at least. I mean, if it all gets too much, I suppose I could leave.'

After four long, gruelling months recovering at home, I felt I was finally ready to return to work. I was dealing with my everyday tasks at home once again – I was on top of my emotions and I'd even recovered my sense of humour. Now when things went wrong, I could laugh. I had the energy to take Betty to the park and play with her properly, and I felt I was more or less myself again.

'You know, before you went off, when it was getting really

bad, I didn't know who was going to walk through that door from one day to the next,' Will said quietly. 'Were you going to come in and bite my head off? Burst into tears? Or just go to sleep? I felt like I was walking on eggshells all the time.'

I checked myself before apologising. I knew this wasn't why Will was telling me this. It wasn't a guilt trip – he was sharing his experience of my depression with me, and it was important for me to understand how badly it had affected him too.

'It's something I've struggled to understand,' I replied thoughtfully. 'How all the stress at work actually affected my whole personality. But it did. I think I spent so long and so much energy trying to hold it in place, it actually consumed me totally. That's the thing – I'm a whole human being. I can't lock different parts of me away and compartmentalise my life. It's just not realistic.'

The time was fast approaching when I knew I had to return to work. Of course, coping at home where there weren't any greater decisions to make than what to cook for tea was one thing. Coping in the tumult of a working day on the labour ward where every small decision was literally a matter of life or death was another. Was I ready? There was only one way to find out.

23

Diving Back In

'Pippa! Welcome back!' Bev greeted me with a huge smile and a massive hug as I walked onto the ward. 'It's so good to see you. How you doing?'

'Yeah, yeah, okay, I think.' I returned her smile, though I was a bag of nerves. It was 7 a.m. on 2 March and my first day back to work after being off for four months with stress and depression. I was as nervous as hell – although I'd managed to throw down a cup of coffee before leaving the house, my stomach was too churned up to eat anything. Then, as I'd pulled into the hospital car park, I looked up at the massive hospital building and had to take several deep breaths to calm myself down. The last time I'd parked here for a day's work I felt out of control, about to explode and on the verge of making an horrific mistake. I recalled that feeling of being so stressed that my brain refused to work properly. It was like being encased in a thick fog. Now the fog had cleared, but would it come back? Would this place consume me again? I steeled myself to get out of the car.

Come on, Pippa, I told myself. *You can do this. You're ready.* Of course, I didn't know that for certain. It was all very well feeling better at home, without any of the day-to-day stresses of the ward, but I needed to stay positive in order to get through the day. I wasn't even this nervous when I went back to work after maternity leave, and that was after a full year away from the ward. Now I would be going back in a 'phased return', which meant I wasn't doing a full twelve-hour day to start with – I would do two weeks of nine-hour days before tackling a full twelve-hour shift.

I have to admit, it was a pretty good start. The moment I walked back onto the ward I was overwhelmed by the warmth and good feeling from my wonderful colleagues. Most of my good friends knew the reason I'd been off, and they were genuinely pleased to see me back. I was so touched by their outpouring I wanted to cry. Meanwhile, Mandy, the coordinator on shift, gave me a hearty 'welcome back', and then invited me to step into a side room with her.

'Pippa, are you alright?' she asked in a concerned voice. I nodded, swallowing back the tears.

'Are you sure you're ready to come back?' she asked seriously.

'Yes, yes, I'm fine,' I said, even as I felt myself welling up.

'I'm serious. Don't come back if you're not ready. The staffing here is diabolical.'

Woah! That wasn't what I expected to hear, but I knew Mandy wouldn't be saying it if she didn't mean it. She was offering me the chance to turn around and walk out again, but if I did that, I knew I would never come back. Was I *really* ready?

Diving Back In

I wavered for a second before replying: 'No, I'm fine. Honestly. I've got to come back at some point.'

'Okay, well, good luck today, and come and find me if you have any problems. But like I said, we're struggling with staffing levels, the worst we have ever been so . . . well, don't say I didn't warn you.'

We went straight into handover with the four other midwives on the ward. I was given a 'grand multipara' to look after, which is a woman who has had more than five children. This lady, Leonie, was only thirty-six years old but this was her eighth pregnancy. She'd given birth to six live babies, all of whom had been taken off her and put into care. Now she was due to give birth again, and this baby too was likely to be taken into care. It's funny, you would expect someone who had lost so many children to Social Services to be anxious about having to give up her next baby, but, according to my colleagues, Leonie was very calm and optimistic. I think she had managed to convince herself that somehow, this time would be different, though we knew from the Social Services notes on her file that there was little chance of her keeping this baby.

Leonie's birth was not straightforward by any stretch. Her baby was an 'unstable lie', which meant he wasn't fixed in the pelvis. In the last few weeks he had been all over the place – he had been both breech (feet down) and transverse (lying across), so as soon as he was head down (cephalic), the doctors decided to break her waters in a controlled environment. This would lower the risk of a cord prolapse. Now, at the same time as I was tasked with looking after Leonie, I was also given a woman in another room who had just delivered her first baby, so there was two hours of paperwork to complete for her.

Okay, I could just manage to keep on top of Leonie, the grand multipara – as well as all the paperwork for the woman who had just delivered – but at 8 a.m. I was given a *third* lady. Kris was coming in for an 'augmentation' – this meant her waters had broken over twenty-four hours earlier but she had not gone into labour. We would need to assess her and then, if her cervix had not yet dilated and was still tight and firm, we would give her a hormone tablet to try and get her going. If that didn't work, we would then put her on the hormone drip. Three women within my first hour back at work! It was madness. Now I was running between three rooms and my head was spinning. I felt panic rising in my chest and, at the same time, a boiling resentment at the stressful situation I'd been put in on my first day back. In my first hour! If I knew who I was meant to complain to, I would have done so, but this was a Saturday and there were no Band 8s around, let alone anyone from HR.

Welcome back. Welcome back! Welcome back! I repeated to myself over and over again, as I trotted between the three rooms, trying to keep all the plates spinning at once.

'I'm sorry,' said Mandy, when she saw me. 'I know it's a lot. As soon as we have somebody free to relieve you, I'll take one of the ladies off you.'

I hadn't expected the management to take it too easy on me on my return – after all, I knew the situation before I went off sick – but this certainly didn't feel like a 'phased return'. This wasn't just throwing me in at the deep end, this was like being towed eight miles off the coast and dumped in the open ocean! If I got through this shift, I knew I could cope with anything. As my anxiety levels rose, I started to experience that same feeling of losing control that I'd had in the weeks leading up to my illness.

It's fine. You're fine, Pippa. It must be because they think you're a really good midwife that they're giving you all this work, I told myself, desperately trying to stop the panic engulfing me.

My first job was to sort out the room of the lady who had just delivered. The place was a complete state, so I changed her bedding, cleaned the blood off the floor, got rid of all the dirty sheets and towels and then sat down to do her paperwork. I put myself on the desk at the end of the corridor, rather than the one in the nurses' station. The desk at the end was much quieter, and if you were in the nurses' station you were bound to find yourself answering phones every five minutes. Everyone was under pressure – today, we were down to six midwives on the birthing unit, and that included the Labour Ward Coordinator. We couldn't even call in the community midwives any more because there weren't any. Our home-birthing service had been suspended indefinitely three months earlier after we'd lost the last of our community midwives and the hospital had failed to replace them.

Fortunately, the morning was calm enough to allow me to complete my paperwork by 10.15 a.m. Then, at 10.30 a.m., Leonie's waters were broken, and from that point she needed continuous monitoring. By 11 a.m. I finally got round to giving the hormone pessary to Kris, my augmentation lady. It was all go, but I managed to stay on top of all three cases without losing the plot. Then, at 12.30 p.m., the lady who had delivered was discharged and I got my first break after five and a half hours. *Phew!* I took myself off the unit, bought a big coffee and sat down in the staffroom for twenty minutes and closed my eyes, just trying to clear my mind and soak up the silence. Being still and quiet, even for just a little while, was exactly what I needed to clear my head and recharge my batteries.

Then, at 1 p.m., I dived back into the fray. At this point, both Leonie and Kris started labouring at the same time.

'Right, I can't do both,' I told Mandy firmly.

'No, of course you can't,' she agreed, checking the board. 'I've got Helen free now so she can take over Leonie and I'll leave Kris with you. That okay?'

I nodded. *This is improving.* By 2 p.m., I'd gone from three ladies down to one. After seven hours on shift, it was the first chance I had to go to the toilet. Half an hour later, Kris was showing signs of an infection. I needed to sort out antibiotics and blood cultures, get her cannulated and bring a doctor on board. I was just checking out some diamorphine for her, when the emergency buzzer went off in theatre. I stopped what I was doing and rushed straight there.

'Flat baby needs resuss,' the registrar announced, as we all piled in.

'Unresponsive baby, not breathing,' the paediatrician now said. 'Heart rate less than a hundred.'

I jumped on the scribe, writing down everything my colleagues were doing and who was in the room. Luckily the baby picked up quickly and was transferred to the neonatal unit. Then I was free to get back to Kris with her diamorphine. Luckily it had only been about twenty minutes, and, since she was a former ITU nurse, she understood when I explained the delay. It was a relief that she was so understanding – some women can get really ratty when you're called away to help with an emergency.

'Where's my pain relief? Where have you been?' they interrogate you. Most will be fairly understanding when you explain that you've been off trying to bring back a lifeless baby, but, even so, it can be very frustrating if someone is in pain and there's a delay in getting them relief. Now it was 4 p.m. – time for me to leave.

* * *

I got back in the car almost in a state of shock. The whole day had whizzed by in what felt like seconds. I suppose that was one thing – I hadn't had time to get too nervous. Driving back home, I didn't know whether to feel elated or exhausted. In truth, I probably felt something of both, and, at the same time, annoyed that absolutely nothing had changed.

'How was it?' asked Will when he got home.

'It's like I've never been away,' I sighed. 'They had me looking after three women from the very start. I honestly thought I was going to go under. I coped somehow, though I didn't really have a choice. There was no time to stop and think. By the time I was down to one lady, I felt a bit more stable.'

'Hmm. Maybe it'll be a bit better tomorrow.'

'Yeah, maybe.'

* * *

But the next day was just as bad. Kris, my augmentation lady, had become septic in the night and had ended up in theatre for a section. Mother and baby were now doing fine,

I was assured during handover, when they were assigned to me. At the same time I was also given a woman on the verge of delivering her second baby. The woman delivered fairly soon after handover, but she had quite a bad tear. I prepared her for suturing, but there was so much blood I couldn't see where the bleeding was coming from. Normally, I would be doing the stitches, but on this occasion, I called the registrar for a bit of support. *Would I have done this before?* I wondered, as she assessed the situation. *Is this really an unusually difficult suture or are my nerves getting in the way?* I couldn't tell. All I knew was that I had to trust my instincts, and my instincts were calling out for more help.

'It's okay, Pippa, I'll do this,' said the registrar, as she prepared for suturing. I thought it would be a matter of moments before it was all done, and I would be thanking her and apologising at the same time for calling her in for such a minor procedure. But the registrar struggled too.

'Yes, I see what you mean,' she muttered, sitting back for a minute to assess the situation again. *Okay, so it's not just me.* In the end she took her to theatre to do it under proper lighting and pain relief. It took her a good hour because the skin was very fragile, and every time she put a stitch in, it tore or broke. Afterwards the registrar confided: 'I've never had to suture a lady like that before. It was one of the hardest I've had to do.'

Just as we were coming out of theatre, the Labour Ward Coordinator flagged me down in the corridor: 'Pippa! Just the person. I've got a lady coming in with your name on her. She wants a pool birth!'

'*Riiiight . . .*' I said slowly, mentally counting up the women

Diving Back In

I now had to look after. 'You do know I've already got the augmentation lady and a perineal tear who's just come out of theatre?'

'Yup.'

'Alright then.'

If I thought day two would be any less stressful than day one I was dreaming. Fortunately, when I admitted the pool lady in triage, she wasn't yet in established labour, so I had at least an hour to concentrate on my perineal tear lady before going back to the pool birth. But two hours later she was 8 cms dilated, and quite rapidly delivered her baby in the pool. I got by, somehow, but it felt like I was flying by the seat of my pants, and all the time I had that sick feeling in the pit of my stomach that an accident could happen at any moment.

The lady who had just come out of theatre needed more attention than I could afford to give. When she'd first come in she had severe pre-eclampsia with blood pressure of 180 over 120. That was stroke level! Fortunately, once out of theatre, her blood pressure stabilised, and she seemed fairly comfortable. Plus, she was incredibly understanding.

'Are you okay? Do you need anything?' I asked hastily, when I managed to get into her room once an hour to do her observations.

'I'm fine, honestly. Don't worry about me.' She smiled, clearly besotted with her newborn baby. Thankfully she had lots of help from her partner and mother, but that didn't stop me feeling guilty. There was no time for a nice, relaxed conversation. No chance to show her how to do the first breastfeed, change her bed linen or her pads. I hovered for one last moment, taking in the scene of this new, very happy family, before I swiftly left the room. I now had five minutes maximum before I had to be on-hand to give the pool lady one-to-one care.

It's not just the aftercare that we're unable to provide. Since I've been back at work, I've discovered a worrying new practice of delaying inductions by twenty-four or even forty-eight hours when we're understaffed. At our hospital, we carry out a maximum of four inductions a day – usually for clinical reasons like pre-eclampsia, gestational diabetes, reduced growth or if the woman has gone two weeks beyond her due date. We usually start them off on the slow release hormone pessary for twenty-four hours before breaking their waters. But it could be that during those twenty-four hours the ward will have to close to elective work because of understaffing. This means the woman can't leave, and we can't break her waters either. We literally have to stop what we're doing for them until the unit opens again (usually twelve hours later). So they remain on our noisy, busy ward, having contractions, getting no sleep, becoming more and more exhausted by the hour. It's not good for the mother and it's not good for the baby. Before now, this was a rarity, but in the last year it's become a regular occurrence.

'I'm sorry, we can't break your waters because there aren't enough midwives on at the moment,' I'll tell the family. 'We've not got anyone to give you one-to-one care, but as soon as a midwife becomes available, we'll go ahead.' They get very frustrated and upset, and it's completely understandable but there's nothing I can do to change the situation. It's stressful for everyone – especially the families who are watching their wife/daughter/partner go

Diving Back In

through this extended process, in pain, when everyone just wants the baby out as quickly and as safely as possible.

* * *

By the end of my first week, I was ready to drop, but I was fairly certain I could cope without falling apart. And that's when the hospital gave me a student midwife to train. *Oh no!* I had begged them not to give me a student during the first month after my return, but that request clearly went straight out of the window.

'Can't you assign her to another midwife?' I asked Jen, as she told me I was now in charge of Bella, a third-year student. Bella was lovely, very sweet. I had nothing against Bella personally, of course, it was just that training a student would put even more pressure on me at a time when I really didn't need it. I had trained plenty of students in the past, but it's not easy. You have to watch them constantly at first, making sure they are capable of basic procedures before teaching them on the job.

'You know the answer to that,' Jen responded dolefully. 'I would if I could.'

And so I took on Bella, a third-year student, only two weeks after I went back to work. That in itself wasn't easy. She lacked confidence. Midwifery university courses have changed since my day, and she had returned from her second-year placement as if she had never been on a ward before.

'I can't do it,' she said, when I asked her to put in a catheter.

'What do you mean? Of course you can, Bella. That's day one, week one. You're just nervous about doing it, that's all. Come on, you can do it. I know you can.'

It was like coaxing a scared rabbit out its hutch. And this rabbit needed a lot of coaxing if I was going to pass her! So, each week I set Bella little goals to bring her skills up to scratch and increase her confidence on the ward. One week her goal might be to increase her multitasking, or improve her supportiveness to the mum; another week she might be tasked with talking to the doctors. At the end of the month, Bella was performing all her tasks much better, and I felt that little bit happier about signing her off. After all, I didn't want to be the senior midwife who failed her, destroying her confidence or her chances of becoming a midwife. In some ways, it was nice to have Bella to focus on, it took my mind off my own worries, but in other ways it was a burden I probably could have done without at a critical time in my career.

Now I was back to work full time, I gradually found myself getting into the swing of things. It was funny – after four months away, I thought that somebody would sit me down at some point for a chat, just to ask me how it was going and whether I was coping. For the sake of not pushing me down the same road again, you'd think the management would have taken a little time and care over my return. But no, there was nothing.

Oh, wait . . . no, that's not true. About two weeks in, I saw Lina.

'Pippa, good to see you back. You alright?' she asked, as she strode importantly down the corridor one afternoon.

'Yeah,' I replied hastily. There wasn't much more I could say, as she didn't actually stop walking. She just kept going as she called out, over her shoulder: 'Good good.' And that was it.

Diving Back In

Six weeks after my return, one of the LWCs shoved a form in my direction and asked me to sign at the bottom.

'What is it?' I asked.

'A "return to work" form, nothing really. A box-ticking exercise. It just says you've had a full debrief, the workload is at safe levels and you feel comfortable and happy. And you commit to not taking any more sick days for the next three months.'

'Oh, right.'

'Yeah, apparently, you should have signed it on your first day back, but, hey ho, it got overlooked. Sorry! If you could just sign here . . .'

And there it was. No acknowledgment for the illness that had driven me out of the ward for four months, no friendly chat to ask me how I felt about the work, nobody asking me if I could cope, or working with me to ensure my future mental good health. Nope, none of that – just a threat to send me to a 'capability meeting' if I had one more day off sick in the next three months. Just one more day. I paused, for a moment on the verge of allowing negative emotions to wash over me, but then I thought back to earlier in the day: the couple who, after years of trying, had finally become a family; the joy of the new mum who had managed to get her baby to latch, and the look between a mother and her baby when I placed him in her arms for the first time. This was never going to be easy, there were still a huge number of hurdles to overcome, but I knew I could do it. So instead I managed a wry smile. *Welcome back, Pippa! Welcome back to the life of an NHS midwife.*

24

Reflections

I still have the letter that Emily gave me – the one where she says that she couldn't have asked for anyone better to walk into the room and deliver her baby. It is one of my most treasured possessions. I recall how my heart swelled with pride when first I read her words, and how much it meant to be acknowledged as 'a fantastic midwife'. I walked a little taller after that day and every day since because, for all the heartache, the stress, the difficulties and pain, I believe that being an NHS midwife is one of the best jobs in the world. It is an honour to be present at the moment a new life is born, and I never forget that. I love my job and I always will, but there is something deeply wrong with a system where the very people who care for others are so badly cared for by their employers.

Today, I'm back at work full time, but it is no thanks to the NHS trust that brought me to my knees. I recovered because I have a wonderful husband who was there for me during those long nights when I cried myself to sleep;

for the days I couldn't speak and for the hours when all I could do was lie in bed watching box sets. Will was there. He listened without judgement, without knowing what to say – sometimes without even knowing what I was really talking about. He just listened and gave me plenty of cuddles afterwards. Then he made me laugh. I got better by going to the park with Betty, taking long walks with the dog, meeting up with my friends, going swimming, doing normal things – in short, just being myself again. I got better because Will told me to write it all down and, in doing so, he found the key to my recovery. Writing allowed me to express my deepest thoughts and feelings without fear of judgement. It allowed me to reconnect with the parts of the job that I love and reminded me why I became a midwife to start with.

In my hospital trust there are no 'thank-yous', no annual reviews, no awards or acknowledgment for the tremendous care and dedication we give to the women and families we look after. And yet, every day I witness overworked and underappreciated staff undertake minor acts of heroism that would make most people weep – it's no wonder that a little note or card from one of the families in our care means so much. We cherish these precious objects as if they are the crown jewels. 'Well done' is not a phrase you hear very often on my ward, but it would certainly improve morale if, once in a while, somebody gave you a little pat on the back. I don't need a cheerleading team to break out into enthusiastic chanting every time I deliver a baby. I know I'm lucky to be in this profession. I know it's a privilege to help a woman give birth, and that in itself is reward enough. But this isn't a 9–5 job. We put our heart and soul into every single delivery. We don't just walk away and put the day behind us. The day follows us home: it comes in our front door, puts its feet up and makes itself very comfortable in front of our TV. Our working day dominates every area of our lives, and that simply can't be helped. After all, this is a vocation for which you give every single fibre of your being. We care about the people we look after and the babies we bring into this world – their health and wellbeing matters to us, even if we have only met them twelve hours before. We are more than just cogs in the NHS machine; each and every one of us is a professional with an individual skill-set and opinions on procedures, practices and performance. If we are to remain a functioning part of the National Health Service, it is absolutely vital that more is done to make all midwives feel more valued by the trust they work for and by the government.

I've seen so many good midwives and healthcare professionals leave my hospital in recent years, either driven out by uncaring practices, or taken to the edge by unrealistic workloads. And, of course, it's always the ones who care the most that fall the hardest. After my recovery, I gradually started to tell people the reason I was off sick. At first, I was embarrassed and ashamed of what I perceived as my personal weakness, but the better I felt in myself, the angrier I became. Why should I be made to carry this shame? It wasn't my fault I went under. And, actually, the more I talked about it, the better I felt. I now tell people quite openly that I am taking antidepressants for stress and depression. What shocks me is the number of people who reply that they too are taking drugs for the same reason. One of the doctors I work with said: 'If I pick five doctor friends at random from this very hospital, at least three of them will be taking antidepressants.' What does that say about how the way the NHS treats its staff? Something is very, very wrong when we are all on chemical mood-enhancers just to get through the working day.

The problem isn't with me; it was never with me. I am still that same 'fantastic' midwife who delivered a sceptical mum's baby fifteen years ago. But I do feel different now. I don't say *yes* to everything. If there is a shortage on the ward, it is a management problem, not mine. Just like I tell Betty I won't clear up the mess she has made, I won't be responsible for their messes either. And yet, the Trust's response to the problem in the form of their 'Resilience Training' programme is not simply inadequate; to me it represents a sinister attempt to shift the responsibility onto individual practitioners. In short, it tells us one thing: if we're feeling stressed, the onus is on us to fix the problem. This completely ignores the fact that the stressful environment is out of our control. That is why we need our unions to stick up for us and be our advocates at a time when we are feeling weak and vulnerable.

According to the Royal College of Midwives, the profession is losing one midwife a day due to the pressures of the job. In England alone, this means almost half of maternity units are turning mothers away each year due to staff shortages. The week I returned to work, our unit was down to six midwives – six midwives for forty-four women! No wonder we're stressed. It's not ourselves we're thinking of; it's the women in our care. We are so overloaded that we can't spend five minutes sitting talking to a new mum, showing them how to do their first feed, or helping them to the toilet.

Reflections

And because of the little things like this, it feels like we're letting them down.

This book is filled with examples of how the NHS funding crisis affects clinical decisions on a hospital ward, and it is clear there are hundreds of different ways this lack of funding negatively impacts upon the standard of medical care. These problems will only worsen until the underlying issues are addressed. Proper funding is a must. And here's a suggestion: we could start by cutting the number of managers in half in order to put the money back into healthcare professionals. I know that sounds simplistic; I know that many clever people will dismiss my suggestion as naïve or impractical. But here's the thing: in my fifteen years as an NHS midwife, the number of managers has doubled while the number of midwives has halved. Meanwhile, I have no idea who my actual line manager is or who I'm meant to complain to if something goes wrong. So while our service is increasingly top heavy, the lines of responsibility have become blurred and there are fewer people actually doing the job. You do the maths.

And the blame game has got to stop. Even though I am back at work, I still fear that one day I'll be summoned to court with no backing from my hospital. Why? If you've been following my story, and my observations on how things have changed for the worse, you have to agree it's because the trusts appear to care more about their own reputation than sticking up for its staff. There is no support or training for dealing with legal cases, but there really should be because they are difficult, stressful and not part of our job description, even though they are becoming increasingly common. On top of that, junior staff keep getting thrown under the bus by senior colleagues, and it really doesn't help make us feel safe and secure in our jobs.

You know, it has always struck me as apt that hospital organisations are called 'trusts'. It is such a small but important word – and to me, it means so much. Trust. When you come through these doors to give birth for the first time, you will put your entire trust in me to help you through this incredible time in your life. And it *could* be me – after all, I'm still working as a midwife in the NHS. I'm still delivering babies daily. I will give you my best possible care, and you will trust me to guide you through the choppy waters of labour, to get you and your baby safely to the other side. Similarly, I put my trust in my colleagues to be there at the moment I need them in a crisis or emergency. I pull my buzzer and I trust they will rush to help. And all of us put our trust in the Trust. We trust that our employers will protect our best interests, defend our work, promote our achievements, respect us as professionals and support our rights. The whole system works because we all trust one another. Trust – it is easily gained but, once broken, so hard to repair.

So perhaps we all need to think about helping midwives and health professionals feel good about the extraordinary work they do. Both as individuals and as a community we need to assign more value and respect to the people who bring new life into this world. It isn't up to just one of us, but all of us. Then we can do the job that we have been trained for, and you can trust us to deliver the next generation. After all, the nation's future is in our hands. We won't let you down.

It is only a year and a half since the hardback edition of this book was published, and yet so much about the world in which we live and work has changed. I am one of the many, many people who work in our wonderful NHS, and each of our experiences in working throughout this pandemic has been unique. But in this next chapter, I want to give you my story in the hope that it sheds light on the reality of working for our health service during these unprecedented times.

25

Covid

I found out first thing in the morning, during handover, that we had our first Covid-positive lady on the ward and that it was me who had been allocated to look after her. I nodded and smiled at my team leader, ready to do my bit and take my turn in the 'red' zone of our ward, but inside I felt sick with anxiety. It was early April 2020 and coronavirus had become our main preoccupation over the last few weeks. I don't think any of us really understood the severity of this new disease until the deaths started creeping up. It wasn't until the end of March that we were all sent for individual fittings for our masks, until then we had carried on as normal – there were no masks on the wards, no testing of patients.

During my fitting I was shown how to put the mask on properly, pressing down on the edges to mould it to the side of my face and nose to seal it. A big hood was then placed over my head, like the type on a beekeeper's suit, and a substance was sprayed inside. If I could taste anything

I was to let them know. It only took a matter of seconds before a bitter, acrid taste filled my mouth and stung the back of my throat. Urgh . . . it reminded me of that stuff my mum painted on my fingernails when I was younger to stop me biting them. The mask hadn't prevented the aerosol droplets from getting through, which meant it had failed.

'It happens,' said the woman doing the fitting. 'This type of mask doesn't suit everyone. But let's try it a second time. Sometimes, it's just a question of getting it really snug.'

On the second try, having not tasted the unpleasant droplets, I passed, and so I was issued with an FFP3 mask – the kind that looks a bit like duck bill – and sent on my way. Still, in the back of my mind I was plagued with doubt. *Had I tasted it after all?* I walked back to the ward, the pungent taste of the droplets still haunting the back of my throat and mouth. A week later we were issued with our Personal Protective Equipment (PPE) and trained in the correct protocols for their use, although it was clear that a number of people had failed the mask test. As a result, staff were wearing all manner of different masks – some had gas masks made from rubber with big tubes on the front and one of my colleagues even wore a sealed hood with a vacuum hose and a battery pack attached to her waist.

Now, as I dressed in my standard-issue PPE, I still felt fearful. The hospital management told us we could rely on this equipment for protection, but would this little mask protect me? Was I putting myself and my family at risk? Trying to push these thoughts from my mind, I moulded the mask tight to my face, pulled on my head visor, climbed into the theatre gown and pulled a pair of gloves over the sleeves before taping them into position. Only once I was sure that every inch of me was covered did I walk through the heavy double fire doors that separated the 'positive' patients from the rest of the ward. Once inside this area I couldn't come out to mix with the other staff so it was just me down here for the rest of the day with our positive mother-to-be.

When I walked into the room I put on my cheeriest smile, at first forgetting about the PPE that almost fully concealed my face. Instead, I hoped she could hear the warmth and care from the tone of my voice, and see it in my eyes. Ayesha sat on the side of the bed, her partner next to her on a chair, and thankfully they both wore masks: though this was not a big room she was already doing a lot of heavy breathing. My eyes slid upwards to the tilted window – well, at least that was open. Now I tried to put coronavirus out of my mind as I set about doing her checks to find out how she was coping.

Ayesha was clearly quite anxious. It was her first baby and the added pressure of having contracted the virus, despite having minimal symptoms, had heightened her uncertainty dramatically. She was still only 2 cms dilated, meaning she wasn't yet in established labour, so I decided to monitor her a bit longer, but after a couple of hours she wasn't much further along, so I made the decision to send her home to establish there. It could be hours yet and while I wanted to give her the best possible care, I knew she might be more comfortable and more relaxed at home.

Ayesha wasn't the only one who was anxious. Every time I went into her room I was conscious of an invisible danger all around. The hardest part was that once I was out of her room, I was alone and it was difficult to distract myself from the rising panic inside my chest. My colleagues were all tucked away behind the fire doors in the 'Covid-negative' ward, where I could hear the reassuring sounds and low-level hum of hospital activity. Here, on my side of the ward, it was deathly quiet. It felt strange and alienating.

That night, I drove home from my twelve-hour shift, trying to recall all the time I had spent with the Covid-positive couple. Had I been careful enough? Had I made sure the mask was pressed tightly around my face? I couldn't afford to take any chances. My mind was still whirring as I pulled up outside my house and went through my 'new' normal routine. First, I took out the antibacterial spray and wipes and wiped down the car seat, steering wheel, gear stick and the car handles. Then, I walked the short distance up the path to our front door. As soon as the door was shut behind me, I took off all my clothes and put them inside a sealed plastic box, then I sprayed the handles of the door and the box and ran upstairs to the shower, careful not to touch a single thing on my way up. In the shower I gave myself a thorough scrub with the foul-smelling antibacterial soap we had recently purchased and washed my hair with shampoo. Putting on some fresh clothes I went downstairs, took the plastic box with my dirty clothes, pulled on elbow-length gloves and loaded the clothes into the washing machine before spraying the gloves with a bleach solution and sanitising my hands one last time.

Out of the corner of my eye I saw my daughter hopping from one foot to the other, almost bursting with excitement. I washed my hands one last time and it was only then, finally, that Betty was allowed to give me a hug. We did this every night but I wouldn't have it any other way. I had to protect my family.

Covid

'Mummy!' Betty flung herself at me, arms wound round my neck. I squeezed her little body tight and covered her with kisses until she giggled and squirmed out of my grasp. She was so good about all our new routines. We had talked to her very early on about coronavirus and like everyone else we had drilled her in the practice and importance of good hygiene and hand washing. She knew that she wasn't allowed to say a proper hello to Mummy until I had been through my 'decontamination' routine because, as she said: 'Mummy needs a shower cos she's got coronavirus on her.'

'Hey there,' Will grinned, handing me a large glass of white wine.

'God, that looks good. Thanks. How was your day here?'

'Great – your clever daughter has done some wonderful maths. You're going to be very impressed . . .'

Since Will's job in film production had stopped overnight he had gone on furlough, which was fortunate since it meant he could stay home with Betty.

'Wow – I'd love to see that,' I nodded enthusiastically, the tightness in my chest from the day's tension slowly beginning to release. 'Go on, darling, go and get your work to show Mummy . . .'

As she scampered out of the room, Will asked me how things had been at work.

'Oh, not bad,' I smiled. 'Usual stuff really . . .'

I didn't tell him about the Covid-positive lady, there was no point making him anxious too. And as long as I had been careful enough everything should be fine . . . Little did I know that this fear and anxiety was to become a part of my daily work routine for many months to come.

The Secret Midwife

During the first wave of the pandemic our hospital trust, like all others up and down the country, made huge changes to our working practices seemingly overnight. We tested everyone who came onto the ward and every woman was treated as positive until they returned a negative test. It slowed everything down, of course, but that couldn't be helped. We had to protect the women, babies and staff on the ward. Partners were only allowed in once a woman was in established labour and all home births stopped immediately. Most people accepted the new rules because we were all going through this frightening time together, though I could see how hard it was for some to let their partners enter the hospital alone, knowing how much pain they were in. Of course the odd one or two got angry and frustrated, especially when rules on mask-wearing were tightened, but when this happened we were very clear about the protocol, telling them that verbal or physical abuse towards staff would not be tolerated. If they still didn't comply, we called Security or occasionally even the police to escort them off the premises. I could totally understand their frustrations but our priority was the safety of our colleagues and the birthing mothers and babies.

But these cases were rare, and the overwhelming feeling we got from the public was that of love and support. We were totally taken aback by the generosity of individuals, families and businesses who organised quickly and started sending in food parcels to the hospital, buying pizzas for the staff, and raising money for moisturisers and hand cream for our very chapped and sore hands. Not to mention the amazingly kind offers of accommodation for those who needed to isolate from their families. It was a terrifying time to work in the NHS but the extraordinary outpouring of goodwill that flooded into our wards every day lifted our spirits.

By the beginning of August staffing was down nearly 50 per cent due to the increasing difficulties of staff having to self-isolate. The Trust's plan to combat the staffing crisis was to limit the number of hospital and GP visits for maternity services by offering a 'we come to you' service and so I temporarily left the hospital to join a community team. It seemed like a brilliant idea and I was all for it. For the first time, I would see women from the start of their pregnancies and, depending on how long this scheme lasted, maybe even all the way through to birth and afterwards, even doing the baby and postnatal checks. It meant I could build up a good, trusting relationship with my birthing women, so they could feel confident about the medical care they were receiving. So now, instead of being in the hospital all day long, I'd work from different GP clinics every day, make home visits for postnatal checks and home births and be on call for hospital admissions when our women went into labour.

From the word go, I loved it. I enjoyed getting to know the women under my care and I especially relished that first magical moment when we listened to the baby's heartbeat together. It is always extraordinary and very emotional. If it wasn't for Covid I would have been the happiest midwife on the planet. But – and it's quite a big but – my new role made me even more vulnerable to the risks of coronavirus. At least in the hospital we had full PPE and a whole area designated as a Covid ward. Going into a dozen houses every week in my standard blue medical mask (we weren't given FFP3s in the community), an apron and a pair of gloves left me feeling rather exposed and anxious.

Jasmine was due to have a planned caesarean at the beginning of September and I'd been seeing her in her GP surgery every couple of weeks over August. We hit it off straightaway, and I always left her appointments with a smile on my face. During her final appointment in the surgery she came in wearing a mask but after a few minutes she said she couldn't breathe so I allowed her to take it off for a minute. After all, I was wearing my mask so I felt protected. Two days later, Jasmine came into hospital for the section and, as per protocol, she was swabbed for Covid before we let her onto the ward. I'd been in that morning to see her and had sat on the end of the bed, talking with her and reassuring her for around forty-five minutes as the usually laid-back and confident Jasmine was understandably now nervous about the upcoming procedure. But a few hours later we got the call – she was positive. My stomach did a little flip. I had been in that room for nearly an hour and all I had on was my apron and a normal mask. I went straight to the washrooms and took a shower. Then I dressed in the full Covid PPE to let her know her result had come back positive and that her C-section would have to be cancelled. Earlier, we had been chatting in just our masks and now I was kitted out in the full garb, telling her she wouldn't be meeting her baby today after all.

As soon as I entered the room in full PPE, I could see her face fall. All the adrenaline and nerves, which had been building as she came closer to the time of the section had been for nothing, 'But I don't have any symptoms . . . ' she said, confused.

314

Covid

'I know, I know. I'm so sorry . . . '

What else could I say? We couldn't take the risk of exposing the whole team, so the section was rearranged for ten days later. And so, having had to mentally prepare herself for the C-section, she now had to deal with being sent home with the thought of doing it all again in ten days. But, of course, babies have their own ideas about timing. Three days later, Jasmine went into labour naturally and was given an emergency C-section, regardless of the Covid!

As her allocated midwife, I went to see her at home after the birth. Jasmine had been in hospital for just a few days, which meant that this was only five days after her positive Covid test and she was most likely still positive. You'd think that in these circumstances the NHS would provide us with adequate PPE for such a high-risk visit, but no! In the community we have nothing more than a thin blue medical mask, a pair gloves and an apron, regardless of who we are visiting. It didn't make any sense to me that I had to wear full PPE in the hospital but I was given nothing more than a thin medical mask in the community – the virus was still the same, whatever the setting! Fortunately, I had also armed myself with a pair of clear glasses that I used on the labour ward, and I put these on to cover my eyes as well. I had planned my visits so Jasmine was the last person on my list, meaning I could go straight home afterwards and take a shower. As I parked up, I steeled myself to enter the two-bedroom flat she shared with her husband and son, neither of whom had been tested. For the next half an hour, I would be sharing a space with potentially three positive cases.

At the front door, I was pleased to see everyone wearing a mask but still, I felt my heart thudding hard in my chest as

I crossed the threshold. *Stay calm*, I told myself. *You have a job to do.* First, I had to check that mum was well, look at the caesarean wound, feel her tummy, and ensure it was healing nicely. Then I had to check over the baby, stripping his clothes off and having a good look to make sure we hadn't missed anything in hospital. I couldn't avoid touching the surfaces so I was sat on the floor with the baby on a changing mat. I had to be as thorough as possible, but at the same time I didn't want to be in that flat a single second longer than was necessary. I kept up my usual friendly patter as I did my work but inside I was panicking. And for the next two weeks I was a mess, terrified about any little sniffle or cough, constantly checking my temperature every other hour and alert to any tiny change in my wellbeing. I even felt myself distancing from my own family, not being as affectionate with Betty until I could be certain the risk was over. Thank God I didn't pick up Covid-19 on that occasion.

At first it felt like there was a lull in pregnant women coming through our doors but the pregnancies rocketed again after last summer. I suppose it was to be expected. What else was there to do when shops, pubs and cinemas were all shut and we were unable to see friends and family?! The women I saw usually fell into two very different camps: either they were very anxious, trying to do everything to minimise their risks of catching Covid, or they just went about their life as before. I understood the anxiety, of course: pregnancy is something that you can't control and coronavirus is yet another element over which you have no control so it makes women feel very vulnerable. And lockdown, isolation and loneliness makes everything harder. They weren't going out and meeting other pregnant women, talking through their experiences, so when they came to us, we had a lot of reassuring to do. I found myself saying repeatedly: 'yes, that's normal', 'don't worry', 'everyone feels like that', 'everything's fine'. But it could be weeks between visits so many pregnant women experienced long periods of worry.

With the exclusion of partners in the pregnancy process, our roles expanded. Since birthing women didn't have anyone else with them at the early appointments or scans, they were more reliant on us as their midwives for emotional support. I only got to meet a partner at thirty-six weeks when I did the birth plans and only then could I reassure them. But they'd waited all that time for reassurance and the lack of contact could make the partner feel disconnected from it all. Often, when they arrived at the birthing ward at the crucial moment in labour, they seemed intimidated and frightened by the rawness of the whole experience. I'd spot them hovering next to the bed, looking lost and uncertain how to help, so I'd try to involve them, suggesting they rub their partner's back or keep them hydrated.

And, perhaps inevitably, with the restrictions on partners in hospital, there were now a lot more women opting for home births. Our Trust restarted home births after the first lockdown ended and we went from around one or two a month to nineteen last November! I do understand this. I think I would be more relaxed at home, knowing my partner and child could be with me throughout. Since the start of my stint in the community, I've attended many home births and I absolutely *love* them. It feels so empowering, helping a woman bring her child into the world in the place she calls home. There are many 'messy moments' when a woman gives birth but there are also moments of such beauty and emotion, and every time I feel really honoured to be part of that important journey.

But, when I have to travel more than the length of a corridor to reach a birthing mother, try as I might, I don't always get there in time. One night I was called at 3 a.m. to attend a home birth an hour away in a completely different city. It was the mother's second baby but her first home birth. Leonie, the other midwife on call covering that area, had already been despatched, but, on the way, I took a call from her on my handsfree.

'I can't find the house,' she wailed. 'It's on a humongous council estate and I'm now sat in a Farm Foods carpark with a flat tyre. I'm stuck.'

'You're joking!'

'No, honestly, I can't move. The husband told me they've put a Trolls duvet outside their door so we know where they are.'

We were one midwife down and the next call was from the husband: 'The contractions are coming really fast, where are you?'

'I'm only ten minutes away . . . I won't be long. The other midwife is a little . . . erm, mechanically challenged at the minute.'

'Okay, she's getting in the pool.'

Five minutes later the husband called again, 'She's pushing, she's pushing . . . '

'Keep breathing, tell her to keep breathing, I'm five minutes away.'

Oh my God. Thank heavens for Google Maps. Still on the phone to the husband, I drove up to what I hoped was the right tower block car park, passing Leonie on the way attempting to change her own car wheel, covered in dirt and muttering under her breath. I waved as I passed. She gave me the finger and I giggled – there was no time to stop and pick her up.

'I can see her! I can see the baby! The head's out!' the husband shouted.

'Brilliant. Just wait for the next contraction.'

'The body's out, the body's out . . .'

'Has baby come then?'

'Yes! No! Nearly, I think!'

I heard him encourage his wife to give one last big push and she screamed.

'She's out!' he shouted. 'She's out and she's a whopper!'

'Good. Lift the baby and give it a really good rub with the towel, make sure baby's alright.'

I held my breath . . . And then I heard it, the sound I'd been waiting for: a sharp bleating cry!

Finally, I parked the car and raced to the entrance hallway of the flats where I saw a Trolls duvet cover outside a front door. I raced up the stairs to find the bedroom where thankfully a healthy baby girl lay on her mother's chest, still in the pool, just seconds old. I did all the checks and was relieved and delighted to find that the baby was fine. Mum and dad were both a bit shocked at the speed of their little girl's arrival, just over an hour tops, but I was thrilled.

'This is free birthing at its best,' I laughed. 'The only thing is, we still have a midwife doing an amazing impression of an RAC mechanic.'

It felt so rewarding to be working in the community, getting to know the women and their families, but Covid has thrown up some difficult complications. One day in

December 2020 I was due to visit a woman who had given birth five days earlier. But as I parked up outside her house I noticed a number of cars in the driveway and, looking through the window, it was obvious there were several adults in the house. I called the woman and asked who was inside. She said it was her mum and dad, aunt, sister and her partner's sister – people from four different households! We were currently in Tier 3 and the law was very clear about indoor mixing.

'Look, I can't come in until you've asked these people to leave,' I said gently. 'I can't put myself at risk and you're putting yourself and your baby at risk inviting these people in.'

'Yeah, yeah, I know . . .' she sighed. 'They just wanted to see the baby.'

'I understand but these are the rules and we have to comply for a reason.'

'Can I take you into a different room? What about if we go upstairs?'

I hesitated. On the one hand I had a duty of care to this woman and her child, on the other hand, going inside this house meant taking an unnecessary risk. She explained that the stairs were right by the front door so I didn't have to walk through the house or encounter anybody before going up. So, reluctantly, I agreed, going to a small room upstairs and performing my work as quickly as possible.

'I shouldn't have come in at all,' I told the young mother.

'I know . . . it's just hard.'

'It's hard for all of us. We're all in the same boat.'

Afterwards, I called my manager – had I done the right thing? I wasn't sure. She said I could have arranged to come

Covid

back at a different time, but, as I pointed out, the blood spot needed to be done on day five.

'Well, you made the right decision for the baby,' she said. 'You provided that care.'

Still, I resented being put in that position. We were all making sacrifices to protect one another and yet here was an example of a family who thought the rules didn't apply to them. My job was to care for that woman and child, but was it really fair to ask me to put my own health at risk to do this?

Fortunately, I've now had my vaccine jab and that has gone a long way to easing my anxiety. I was so grateful to be vaccinated, it meant I could finally start enjoying my job again, helping bring babies and joy into the world without fear of catching a deadly virus. The fact is, I'm not a hero. All I ever wanted was to do the job I love and to be protected from harm while doing it. I never volunteered to put my life on the line in the process. And I think that goes for a great many of us – midwives, hospital porters, supermarket workers, postal workers, bus drivers, delivery drivers – all of us who have worked on the frontline during this pandemic.

We're not heroes. We're just like you. If this crisis has shown us anything it is that we're all the same underneath, sharing the same hopes, dreams, vulnerabilities, pain, fear, stress and aspirations. And all our actions affect one another. In our communities we rely so much on the person next to us doing the right thing. I hope that out of this horrible experience we can learn to take care of each other better, and rebuild a kinder, more caring society, one that looks after the frail, the sick, the vulnerable and the people who look after us. You can be sure I'll be here every day, doing my bit for every mother and child in my care.

Glossary

Abruption – when the placenta is pushed away from the uterine wall

Amniotic sac – bag of fluid inside a uterus where the unborn baby develops and grows. Sometimes called the 'membranes' because the sac is made of two membranes called the amnion and the chorion

Bakri balloon – device that inflates with water to put pressure on the inside of the uterine wall to stop bleeding

Bradycardia – when a baby's heartbeat slows right down and takes time to get back up again

Cholestasis – an increase in bile acids in the blood, causing a woman to itch on her hands, feet and abdomen. This is a potentially life-threatening condition because the acid in the blood can cause the baby to go into cardiac arrest

Glossary

Cool Cot – a cot that is temperature controlled to aid preservation of a deceased baby

Cord prolapse – when the umbilical cord shoots down birth canal and presents before baby has emerged

CTG (cardiotocography) technical means of recording the foetal heartbeat and uterine contractions

Descendance – movement of the baby down the birth canal

Embolization – method of treating gynaecological haemorrhage in a variety of clinical situations, including postpartum haemorrhage, bleeding after caesarean section and bleeding following gynaecological surgery

Hypoxia – dangerous condition in which the body, or a region of the body, is denied adequate oxygen supply. This is a common complication in newborn pre-term babies whose lungs aren't fully developed

Intubation – neonatal endotracheal intubation (ET) refers to the placement of an endotracheal tube (breathing tube) within an infant's airway. It is a commonly needed and potentially life-saving intervention for infants both following birth and during neonatal intensive care

Meconium – newborn faeces composed of materials ingested during time spent in the uterus. Unlike later faeces, it's viscous, usually being a dark olive green

Occiput posterior (or OP position) – when the back of the baby's head is lying against the mother's back in utero

Pinard – older-style handheld metal horn for listening to baby's heartbeat that predates the Sonicade (see below)

Polyhydramnios – an excess of waters

Pre-eclampsia – pregnancy complication characterised by high blood pressure and signs of damage to another organ system, most often the liver and kidneys. Pre-eclampsia usually begins after 20 weeks of pregnancy in women whose blood pressure had been normal. Left untreated, preeclampsia can lead to serious and even fatal complications for mother and baby

Sonicade – small handheld device use to listen to a baby's heartbeat (see also Pinard)

Tachycardia – rapid heart rate of baby in the womb

Ventouse delivery – an assisted birth where a suction cup is used to help deliver the baby

Ventouse suction cup – a soft or hard plastic or metal cup that is attached to baby's head to assist delivery